ROUTLEDGE LIBRA
HEALTH, DISEASE

Volume 8

THE FAMILY LIFE OF
SICK CHILDREN

THE FAMILY LIFE OF SICK CHILDREN

A Study of Families Coping with Chronic Childhood Disease

LINDY BURTON

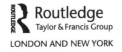

Routledge
Taylor & Francis Group

LONDON AND NEW YORK

First published in 1975 by Routledge & Kegan Paul Ltd.

This edition first published in 2022
by Routledge
4 Park Square, Milton Park, Abingdon, Oxon OX14 4RN

and by Routledge
605 Third Avenue, New York, NY 10158

Routledge is an imprint of the Taylor & Francis Group, an informa business

© 1975 Lindy Burton

British Library Cataloguing in Publication Data
A catalogue record for this book is available from the British Library

ISBN: 978-0-367-52469-2 (Set)
ISBN: 978-1-032-25861-4 (Volume 8) (hbk)
ISBN: 978-1-032-25877-5 (Volume 8) (pbk)
ISBN: 978-1-003-28539-7 (Volume 8) (ebk)

DOI: 10.4324/9781003285397

Publisher's Note
The publisher has gone to great lengths to ensure the quality of this reprint but points out that some imperfections in the original copies may be apparent.

Disclaimer
The publisher has made every effort to trace copyright holders and would welcome correspondence from those they have been unable to trace.

The family life of sick children

A study of families coping with chronic childhood disease

Lindy Burton

Nuffield Department of Child Health,
The Queen's University of Belfast

Routledge & Kegan Paul
London and Boston

First published in 1975
by Routledge & Kegan Paul Ltd
Broadway House, 68-74 Carter Lane,
London EC4V 5EL and
9 Park Street,
Boston, Mass. 02108, USA
Set in 10/12 English
and printed in Great Britain by
The Lavenham Press Ltd, Lavenham, Suffolk
© Lindy Burton 1975

ISBN 0 7100 8171 5 (c)
0 7100 8172 3 (p)

For my parents, with love and gratitude

Contents

Tables

Acknowledgments

Few studies could be completed without much general goodwill, and this is no exception. Mothers, fathers and sick children devoted hours of leisure time to answering my questions, and their patience and kindness made my task a most rewarding one.

Similarly, I am indebted to the Cystic Fibrosis Research Trust, which not only provided financial assistance for this project, but also through the enthusiasm of its members, most especially its Executive Director, Ron Tucker, supplied an unfailing source of encouragement.

To my paediatric colleagues I am indebted for access to patients, and I am especially grateful to Dr John A. Dodge who completed physical assessments on all the children concerned. My thanks are due also to Professor Ivo J. Carré for his constant interest in the study, to Dr and Mrs Garth McClure for their useful comments, and to Dr K. D. MacRae of the Department of Medical Statistics, The Queen's University, Belfast, who offered advice and practical help at each stage in the statistical analysis of results. To Mrs Marilyn McKee and Miss Brenda Sloan I am indebted for the many hours of hard work which they put into the typing of this book.

Finally I am immensely grateful to Virginia and Jonathan who endured the process of creation with such good humour.

Introduction: Sick children and their parents

This is a book about chronically sick children—their fears, their hopes, and the ways in which they face up to their illness. It is also a book about their parents—the problems and difficulties which beset them, and the ways in which they manage to transcend these.

Until quite recently such a book would have seemed an irrelevance. In previous generations childhood scourges were common and medical knowledge and social standards were such that little could be done to control disease. Once contracted, fatal illnesses tended to be brief and infant and child mortality were correspondingly high. Thus saving life was the sole and essential priority for all those concerned with the care of sick children. Naturally, in such circumstances, the physical needs of the patient were paramount. His social and emotional needs were largely overlooked.

Fortunately, this is no longer true today. Over the past fifty years improvements in domestic hygiene, nutrition, and living standards, together with considerable extensions in medical knowledge have significantly improved the health and life expectancy of our population.[1] Many previously crippling conditions are controlled and most

---

[1] Mortality in childhood is highest during the first year of life. Taking the infant mortality rate (number of deaths per 1,000 live births) for the United Kingdom one sees that the infant death rate has now fallen to one-tenth of the level observed at the turn of the century, for instance:

Between
$$\left. \begin{array}{ll} 1906\text{-}10 & 117\cdot1 \\ 1926\text{-}30 & 67\cdot6 \\ 1946\text{-}30 & 36\cdot3 \\ 1956\text{-}60 & 22\cdot6 \\ 1966\text{-}70 & 18\cdot4 \end{array} \right\}$$
 infants died in the first year of life

Figures taken from the Statistical Review of the Registrar General for England and Wales, Year 1970).

infectious diseases have assumed manageable proportions.[1] Now not only are more children likely to survive childhood, but, by contrast to former generations, they are less likely to be ill during their lifetime.

Progress such as this is cause for rejoicing—both for its own sake, and because it conveys the additional advantage of liberating caring personnel from the need to concentrate solely on reversing symptoms. Consequently, in recent years, interest in the whole child—and most especially his emotional and social needs—has escalated.

Much early work in this area can be attributed to the sensitive observations of psychoanalytically orientated clinicians. Recognising the importance of the child's fantasy world in terms of his personality development, they were swift to appreciate the apprehensions of young children faced with threatening events such as hospitalisation (Bowlby, 1971, best summarises the early literature), surgical procedures (Pearson, 1941), and immobilisation (Bergmann, 1945). The anxieties attendant on various chronic or fatal diseases were also explored (Bruch and Hewlett, 1947; Dubo, 1950; Morrow and Cohen, 1954; Josselyn *et al.,* 1955; Schoelly and Fraser, 1955; Natterson and Knudson, 1960). Similarly, it was perceived that childhood fears gradually evolved, being produced initially in response to separation, later by threat of injury, and finally by thought of death (Nagy, 1948, 1959; Solnit and Green, 1963; Green, 1967; Waechter, 1968; Hogan, 1970; Burton, 1971). It became obvious that such fears could affect and prolong the illness (Blom, 1958) and ultimately diminish the young patient's will to live, seriously limiting his willingness to participate in treatment programmes (Langsley, 1961). As a result, many paediatricians stressed the need for creating a 'climate of security' in which the sick child could function most effectively (Howell, 1963; Saunders, 1969; Lawson, 1971).

This need would seem increasingly essential. From all sides there comes news of improvements in life expectancy for children with illnesses which only ten years ago would have proved swiftly fatal. Cancer, leukaemia, and cystic fibrosis (the subject of this present

---

[1] The decline in child mortality due to infections is equally marked. In 1931 over 2,000 children per million living, aged 1-14 years died of infectious disease in the United Kingdom, as compared to under 100 for a similar population in 1970. (Figures taken from S. R. Meadow and R. W. Smothells, *Lecture Notes on Paediatrics,* Blackwell, Oxford, 1973, p. 249).

study) are all yielding to research endeavours and improved treatment techniques (Edelstyn, 1974; Till *et al.*, 1973; Dobbs, 1970). Sick children thus affected may now live for many years. Consequently, as life is extended the problem of maintaining such children in a normal happy state is both growing in size and complexity. Not only are more sick children continuing to live, albeit on constant treatment, but each individual patient is also being faced with the task of coping with his illness over a much longer period. In such circumstances it becomes crucial to review the quality of the life provided. There would seem little value in offering good quality physical life if one cannot also offer viable psychological survival. This then is the prime task of those who care for sick children, and to fulfil it they must both comprehend the emotional and social stresses which the disease creates for the child, and formulate a policy of support and reassurance, which takes account of the child's own instinctive coping strategies.

The child is not alone in his plight—his illness, and his reactions to it, undoubtedly affect his parents. In turn their reactions affect the child, colouring his approach to the disease, therapy, and life in general. It is clearly essential therefore to understand the parent's reactions in the situation.

As yet little is known of the responses of fathers to their child's illness and this present study is perhaps a first tentative step in that direction. However, several clinicians have considered the impact of the child's disease on his mother and many attendant anxieties and apprehensions have been noted (Bozemann *et al.*, 1955; Orbach *et al.*, 1955; Tisza, 1960; Natterson and Knudson, 1960; Cummings *et al.*, 1966). The mother's attitudes to the child seem important both in the causation of certain psychosomatic states (Burton, 1968, summarises some early literature) and also in the extension of more chronic conditions (Bruch and Hewlett, 1947; Green and Solnit, 1964). Where her attitudes are faulty or where marital disharmony prevails, the child's functioning—emotional and physical—is correspondingly limited.

Parents do not exist in an emotional vacuum and many pre-existing factors shape their attitude to illness and the task of rearing a handicapped child. The attitudes of their other children, their own parents, and extended kin may be important determinants of their behaviour (Friedman *et al.*, 1963; Friedman, 1967; O'Connor and Knorr, 1968; Haller, 1970; Debuskey (ed.), 1970; Walker *et al.*,

1971). Background factors existing even prior to the establishment of the family, such as social class membership, ethnic origins, religious affiliation and financial status, may also mould the way in which they cope with the task of rearing a chronically sick or handicapped child (Jordan, 1962; Hewitt with Newson, 1970; Freeston, 1971). Other factors important to a full understanding of family functioning are the age of the child at the onset of symptoms, his sex and birth order, the severity of his illness state, the phenomenal aspects of the illness, the parents' previous personalities, the prior losses sustained by them, the special meaning the sick child has for them, and the support they can offer each other (Tisza, 1960). To understand the reactions of parents in the situation one must therefore know a great deal about them.

It has long been recognised that the strain of rearing a chronically sick child can precipitate family disintegration. Equally it has been recognised that effective patient and parent functioning can occur, and many writers have gained the impression of family strength rather than weakness in the face of adversity (Henley and Albam, 1955; Chodoff et al., 1964; Hewitt with Newson, 1970; McCollum and Gibson, 1971). Indeed some studies have gone further in suggesting that illness—albeit chronic—can improve parent-child relationships, making for better personality functioning on both sides (Bergmann, 1965; Jabaley et al., 1970). In such circumstances the parents are somehow enabled, despite their own often considerable fears and worries, to continue functioning effectively as parents. In addition they seem able to assist the child to keep his 'distress within manageable limits' (Visotsky et al., 1961). The processes by which this is done are still not clearly understood. Perhaps the secret lies in a combination of maintaining a sense of hope, emphasising the child's own personal worth, and encouraging him to use his intact faculties, thereby transcending his infirmity. Such a positive approach is not only important to attitude and life style, but also to the progress of the disease, for as one clinician has emphasised: 'If a child can become convinced that his disability is only relative, half of the therapeutic battle is won' (Haller, 1970). As yet almost no assessments have been made of the factors which maximise positive coping behaviour on the part of either the young patient or his parents. A few tentative conclusions have emerged from a recent study (Stacey et al., 1970) but they refer only to the response to hospitalisation of young children, and do not deal with the immensely greater problem of the parents and child coping with a chronic, and possibly life-shortening, condition.

Because of the scarcity of work in this area, and also because of the immeasurable importance of isolating factors which contribute both positively and negatively to the sick child's wellbeing it was decided not only to undertake this present study, but also to accord especial attention within it to the coping strategies utilised by all family members when living with a chronic childhood disease.

1

Children with cystic fibrosis

This is a study of the family life of one very special group of sick children—children suffering from cystic fibrosis. This disease is inherited—in fact, it is the most common inherited disease in north-west Europe—with one in every twenty of us carrying the faulty gene which produces the disorder. Despite this, until recently, most people had never heard of cystic fibrosis.[1] In one sense this was not surprising. The disease was only detected in 1939, and knowledge of it was slow to spread. For many years children suffering from cf went undiagnosed, being labelled 'delicate' or 'chesty'. Until the advent of antibiotics, little was available to counteract the lung infections which form the scourge of this disease, so even children correctly assessed as suffering from cf could not benefit from adequate medication. As a result few cf children lived much beyond infancy, and most died long before school age with symptoms resembling gastroenteritis or pneumonia.

Fortunately in the past ten years diagnostic procedures have become more accurate, and treatment has improved, with the result that more affected children are being detected early, before crippling physical damage can occur, and, when given adequate preventive treatment, live longer. Because of this, interest has begun to focus on the quality of life provided for the sick child and his parents, and research studies such as this, have gone beyond therapy and

[1] Hereafter abbreviated to cf.

diagnosis, to include the social and psychological wellbeing of the child and his family.

Basically cf presents the child with numerous problems. Because the disease produces a thickening of the mucus throughout the body, many of the child's internal organs become blocked. This affects different children in different ways, though most children have trouble with their lungs. Whereas normal mucus is thin and slippery, and helps in the expulsion of germs and dust, the mucus produced by cf tends to gum up the breathing tubes, leading to infection and lung damage. As a result, many cf children have difficulty breathing. They wheeze, choke, or emit constant irritating coughs. When they try to run or exert themselves they have insufficient breath, and have to stop and choke. Whilst frequently present from earliest days, and often producing vomiting in the baby and young child, such problems become most noticeable and most distressing for the school-age child who is expected to participate in team games, or take part in the normal rough and tumble of everyday play. In every way the cf child is disadvantaged, being slower in running than his well peers, having to pause often to cough, and being unable to clamber easily over obstacles or equipment. Thus often cf children fall behind in play, choosing increasingly younger companions.

The sticky mucus tends also to block the tiny ducts from the child's pancreas, thereby preventing an adequate flow of enzymes into the child's digestive tract. This leads to poor absorption of food, especially of fats. As a result, cf children, if left untreated, fail to put on weight or thrive, despite a normal intake of food. Instead they remain frail and skinny, and pass large, foul-smelling, bulky motions. Naturally these physical attributes do nothing to add to the child's self-esteem, and, with increasing age, many cf children remark disparagingly on their smallness and apparent frailty, both of which are additional obstacles to full participation in normal rough and tumble.

In extreme cases the mucus can be so thick that a blockage occurs in the child's intestines in the first days of life, requiring immediate surgery. This not only puts a strain on the infant and his parents, but produces scars which can be a source of embarrassment in later years.

As yet no cure is available for cystic fibrosis, and children born with it need constant care. In addition, both they and their parents are haunted by the realisation that without such care the child may die. Cystic fibrosis can still prove fatal, and indeed ranks third after accidents, and malignant diseases, as a killer in childhood. To counter this possibility the cf child requires vigorous treatment, beginning as early as possible, preferably before any lung damage has occurred. Replacement enzymes are needed with every meal so that the sick child can better digest his food. Special diets or extra vitamins may be required to help him grow, and antibiotics are given either intermittently or continuously to combat lung infections. In addition, every cf child must have physiotherapy twice or thrice daily to help expel the sticky mucus from the lungs, and some children may need to sleep in a special tent, which is filled with dampened air, so that they can breathe more easily. All this treatment is normally given in the child's own home and has to be provided by the parents. Obviously such an extensive programme challenges even the most able. It also adds to the cf child's sense of difference. As he grows he becomes increasingly aware of the fact that other children do not live as he lives, and it is not long before he wants to know why.

Besides these many illness symptoms, and their counterbalancing treatments, cf children and their parents have to contend with swift and often unexpected changes in the child's physical state. One day a cf child may seem in normal health, the next day he may be grappling with a lung infection or a bowel blockage. Hospitalisation may be imperative. Fortunately not all children are severely affected. Considerable individual differences are apparent both in the degree to which children are affected by the illness and also in the type of symptoms which predominate. Some children may be quite mildly affected, and lead lives almost indistinguishable from normal, others are truly invalided.

Cystic fibrosis compared with other chronic diseases of childhood

Whilst it may be argued that the number of children suffering from cf is relatively small,[1] none the less, in many ways cystic children typify children suffering from other more common disorders. A consideration of their difficulties and problem-solving techniques

---

[1] Aproximately 1 child in every 1,600 is born with cf in the United Kingdom, so that approximately 400 new cases occur every year.

can, therefore, assist those interested in the welfare of other handicapped children.

Inevitably cf involves parents in an extensive home-based treatment programme. The work load is considerable. Thus families coping with cf closely resemble families coping with physical handicaps such as spina bifida or cerebral palsy,[1] or, indeed, mental handicaps such as mongolism.[2] Whilst the actual care required is somewhat different, the encroachment on parental leisure, and the drain on parental energies is much the same. Similarly, mothers of all these children may find themselves unable to accept outside employment because of the need to care for their handicapped child, or to arrange and fit in with special schooling facilities.

Cystic children require regular medication, and frequently some alteration in their diet. In this they closely resemble many other chronically ill children. For example, diabetics require regular administration of insulin, asthmatics require preventive inhalations, coeliacs a cereal-free diet, and phenylketonuriacs a diet free from phenylalanine. Although the actual therapeutic agents and dietary regimes are different, the end product in terms of the child and his parents is a regularity of life, an increased interest in bodily functions and a limitation of freedom.

Cystic children often require emergency hospitalisation to combat lung infections and bowel blockages. Similarly asthmatics are admitted to hospital when an attack becomes too severe to be dealt with at home. Haemophiliacs also require hospital admission whenever bleeding cannot be controlled. Such hospitalisation increases parental anxiety and can diminish the child's self confidence, contributing to emotional difficulties, both at the time and subsequently.

These problems put strain on the parents of cystic children. In addition, as with parents of spina bifida, mongol, phenylketonuriac and haemophiliac children, they are disturbed by the knowledge that their child's disease is inherited. The pattern of inheritance, and the risk of repetition differ, but the sense of guilt and responsibility is constant. These parents are further strained by the need to consider family limitation.

[1] Cerebral palsy occurs at the rate of approximately 1 in every 300 live births in the United Kingdom.

[2] Mongolism occurs at the rate of approximately 1 in every 600 live births in the United Kingdom.

As emphasised previously, until recently cf carried a very high risk of early mortality. Now, fortunately, this risk has been reduced and the outlook for affected children is increasingly better. Nevertheless, there is still no cure for cf, and without proper treatment it can prove fatal. Parents, appreciating this, are forced to accept the possibility of losing their affected child long before such loss should occur. They must, therefore, live through a process of anticipatory mourning, and adjust their expectations accordingly. Thus they closely resemble the parents of children suffering from some, as yet incurable, forms of cancer and leukaemia. Whilst the outlook for such children is also improving, these diseases are still potentially fatal and parents must adapt to this fact. In all these cases the parents' consequent emotional and physical distress is both considerable and long-lasting.

Previous studies of families coping with cf

Few systematic studies of cf families exist, though some sketchy descriptions and fragments of information concerning such families have appeared in social work and medical journals during the past decade. Generally these early reports suffer from a lack of exactness. Social and psychological problems observed in cf patients and their families are attributed solely to the disease, and few attempts are made to evaluate other potentially causative factors, such as previous distortions in the personality of the individuals concerned, or financial and social pressures not directly related to the illness. No incidence is given of the problems observed, rather it is usually implied that all patients and their parents suffer equally. But this is not so. Considerable individual differences do exist. Whilst some families are truly crippled by their experiences, others emerge largely unscathed or even strengthened. The early studies, by over-generalising, mask these differences, and therefore obscure one essential aspect of the problem, that is, the factors which make for strength or weakness in the face of chronic disease.

Similarly, few early studies attribute any significance to cultural factors in shaping family attitude to cf. Yet cultural, racial, and socio-economic differences are vitally important determinants of family attitudes and behaviour. Even the presence or absence of economic help for families of handicapped children may have a profound effect on the ability of such families to contend with the emotional stresses involved. The sadnesses implicit in rearing a chronically sick child are undoubtedly compounded when parents have to sacrifice their own comforts, and those of their well children, to provide medicines, equipment and hospital care for their sick child. Such financial stresses naturally colour the parents' attitude to the disease, and their behaviour both towards the sick child, and the clinicians who care for him. Little attention is paid to such factors in the early studies, yet many of them emanate from states in which little government help is available to assist affected families. This may further explain the essentially negative tone of earlier reports.

It would be wrong to dismiss the findings of these earlier studies too swiftly, however. Despite the inadequacies noted, most concur in their descriptions of the social and psychological problems associated with cystic fibrosis. This concurrence gives them a corporate strength, and they therefore form a useful introduction to the study of the effects of cf on a family.

The first work was done by Turk (1964), a Maryland social worker, who emphasised the financial burdens placed on the parents of a cf child in her state, and noted a resulting 'undercurrent of apprehension and stress'. She found parents deprived of time and energy, and noticed communication problems both between married partners and parents and children. She concluded that many cf children were locked in a 'web of silence', believing themselves an enormous burden on their family.

Two years later, a team of Canadian paediatricians (Lawler, Nakielny and Wright, 1966) commented on the parents of eleven affected children attending their cf clinic. Noting 'marked intra-psychic and interpersonal conflicts' amongst them, they found eight mothers to be clinically depressed and 'living in the shadow of death'. 'Most' (no exact incidence was given) mothers demonstrated repressed hostile feelings to the children for being a burden on them. Fathers showed 'unusual evidence of psychopathology'—one being grossly psychotic, one paranoid alcoholic, and three having peptic ulcers which the authors deemed reactive to the wives' preoccupation with the child's illness. In six families the marital relationship was so severely strained that separation was considered. Not surprisingly, cystic children reared by these stressed couples were markedly anxious, 'preoccupied with death', had depressive feelings, frequent crying spells, and a 'sense of foreboding or impending catastrophe'. Whilst all the children were average or above average in intelligence, the majority were found to be underfunctioning in terms of school achievement.

Before one accepts these conclusions it is well to remember that the sample was very small, and quite possibly a selected one. Also, the families were seen in a psychiatric clinic, which may have added to their apparent discomfort. In addition, no evidence was presented to support the assumption that illness alone caused these psychiatric disturbances. They may have existed prior to the birth of the cystic child, and merely been exaggerated by it. Marital tensions in the parents and disturbed personality growth in the children might, therefore, be more properly attributable to the parents' pre-existing personality problems, rather than to the impact of cf on the family. None of these possibilities was explored by the authors, nor was any attempt made to evaluate the effect of financial and other practical stresses on the parents' ability to cope with the disease.

Comparable deficiencies were found in a study by Cummings *et al.* (1966). Working in Chicago, and using a battery of psychological tests, they found that the mothers of chronically ill (including cf) children showed higher levels of psychological discomfort and social disorientation than mothers of normal children. This they attributed solely to the illness, without reference to the more general economic problems which illness posed for a family in their community. Similarly Kulczycki *et al.* (1969) ignored economic factors when noting 'anger', 'many complicated feelings', a great deal of anxiety, and in some cases a 'conscious rejection of the child' among mothers of twenty-six cf children they studied. Like Turk, these authors found that all families experienced varying degrees of discomfort when talking about cf between themselves or with the child, and they also noted 'little or no discussion of feelings' between spouses. To some extent the lack of parent-child communication may be explicable in terms of the youth of the children concerned. All were under ten, a third were under three. Most parents would find it hard to discuss such a complex disease with such young children.

Whilst Kulczycki and his colleagues initially attributed all these difficulties solely to the impact of cf on the family, Kulczycki (1970) later redressed the balance by emphasising the 'enormous expense' involved in providing paediatric care for a cystic child in the USA. Whilst noting that in some American states the Crippled Children's Program is taking over much of the financial burden, none the less, he found that the cost was still 'prohibitive to the majority' of parents. In nearly a third of the states a family was still forced to meet the total treatment cost unaided. To a great extent financial stresses must exaggerate parental anxiety, increasing the children's distress. Understandably, therefore, as Turk (1964) observed, cystic children in the USA must rightly feel a financial burden on their parents.

This point was also made by McCollum (forthcoming) who found that 79 per cent of fifty-four cf families in Connecticut had one parent or both taking on extra work to provide necessary additional income to pay for the cost of medical treatment. 'Therefore opportunities for gratifying marital interactions were reduced and the parents seldom enjoyed an evening out together.' Even with one affected child, 'Such a family was confronted with the depleting financial drain of the illness—including paramedical expenses the total amount equaling nearly a quarter of such a family's low moderate income.' Yet most of these children were ineligible for help under the Crippled Children's Aid Program, and only one-quarter had sufficient private insurance cover to meet the bulk of hospital costs.

In the circumstances it is not surprising to find considerable family distress, occasioned by cf, in the USA. There the disease is not only a physical handicap, but also an overwhelming financial burden, which understandably produces marital, social and psychological problems. Such difficulties are also found in other non-welfare states, for example two Australian workers (Beveridge and Lykke, 1973) also noted the considerable financial stress which parents of cf children sustain in their community. As a result they argued for greater government support to meet such costs.

But cf poses other social problems for parents, not least those encountered in understanding and coming to terms with the disease. Rosenstein (1970) noted the bewilderment experienced by some parents when first told the diagnosis, and suggested that cf, being relatively unknown, may be viewed as a socially unacceptable disease, such that parents may be reluctant to discuss it with anyone, even the patient. Rosenstein remarked on the overwhelming burden of caring for several affected children, and the near impossibility for parents of maintaining optimism when watching a later-born cf child recapitulate the course of a previously deceased sibling. Also, like Lawler *et al.* (1969) and Turk (1964) he noted marital problems, which he attributed to stresses inherent in rearing a chronically sick child.

Perhaps the most careful American study was that completed by McCollum and Gibson in Yale (1970). Using information gleaned from questionnaires, psychiatric social work interviews, and monthly parent group meetings, the authors saw a pattern in the cf families' problems. Initially, in the prediagnostic stage, parents were faced with the problem of obtaining an adequate and accurate diagnosis. Mistrust of, and hostility towards, medical personnel could be engendered if incorrect diagnoses were made. Often early mother-child relationships were characterised by self-doubt, self-reproach and outright hostility. When the diagnosis was made, parents experienced 'an acute anticipatory mourning reaction' and mobilised psychic defences to 'ward off recognition of the child's danger', such as disbelief, denial, lack of feeling and repression. At a later stage, when parents began to accept the significance of the diagnosis, the feeling components of anticipatory mourning were noted, and parents suffered sleep and appetite disorders and intense grief. Guilt and anger were also noted. At a final stage, that of long-term adaptation, the problem was that of 'maintaining a relationship with a potentially dying child' which afforded some parental gratification and fulfilled the child's physical and psychological needs. 'This stage was characterised by a fluctuating balance between intercurrent mourning and denial of prognosis.'

By contrast to the early American studies, which stressed the problems for parents arising from cf, those coming from Britain emphasised the child's responses to his illness. In 1966, Batten described how cf teenagers rebel against undue parental over-protection, and he drew attention to the fears engendered in some adolescent patients whose growth spurt was delayed. In the same year, Edwards wrote of the older child's fears when hospitalised. She described his apprehensions regarding his health, his inability to participate in social activities with his friends, and his concern over interrupted school work.

Their observations were paralleled by a descriptive study of twenty-one cf children (three to sixteen years) emanating from Duke University Medical Centre. The authors (Spock and Stedman, 1966) assessed the children's progress in a paediatric outpatient clinic, after a routine clinic visit for medical and physiotherapeutic treatment—not perhaps the best milieu for relaxed, informal discussions!

They found the children anxious, and expressing feelings of inadequacy and a need for support. They noted an 'anxious verbal output' during the interviews and concluded that the cf child expressed his anxiety by becoming 'more highly verbal'. Similarly his anxiety could be expressed by 'politeness, neatness and social conformity'.

Extrapolating from these findings, and comparable descriptions of children with malignancy, Pinkerton (1969) argued that paediatricians may be 'in danger of condemning our most advanced cases to a comfortless state of utter loneliness, cut off from emotional communication, consumed with fear of the unknown, the victim of agonizing doubts'—in short subjecting them to the 'web of silence' observed by Turk (1964). To prevent this, Pinkerton argued for a 'partnership of candor' between the physician, the parents and the child. Such a partnership was absolutely essential with the older child, who might 'correctly interpret pandering by parents as of ominous import and draw his own conclusions. In so doing he becomes increasingly dispirited and disconsolate thus endangering his will to persevere with the vital program of therapy.' As a result, Pinkerton believed that 'the child's general resistance can be proportionately lowered, and an insecure doubt-ridden child, or adolescent, is not in an optimum state of health to combat cystic fibrosis'.

Emphasising this crucial link between morale and response to therapy, Teicher (1969) reported renunciation of all treatment routines by lonely adolescent cf patients, who declared their wish to die quickly. He reported suicide attempts by overdoses of medication or sedatives, and concluded that such patients were 'depressed, angry, feel hopeless, helpless and isolated by virtue of their illness'. In addition, he stated 'some parents give the message "I wish you were dead". Many young people oblige.'

Tropauer et al. (1970) also found that depression could seriously impair a cf child's physical progress. He and his colleagues noted 'feelings of inadequacy or insecurity or both' in 75 per cent of the drawings of the twenty cf children they studied, and they noted that the child's early memories and dreams were punctuated with themes of illness, injury, and hospitalisation. One third of the mothers said their cf child had voiced concern about dying prematurely. This was especially true of teenagers. Disciplinary problems, excessive dependency, over-sensitivity and shame about cf, were also noticed.

Tropauer found that 'such concerns were more frequently seen in families where the parents lacked the ability to face the situation openly and rely upon one another for emotional support'.

Thus, 'in families where children were unco-operative with therapy or ashamed of their illness the situation was often characterised by marital difficulties, lack of closeness and harmony or inability of the parents to handle their anxiety by open and supportive communication with each other and their children'. By contrast 'where openness and mutual support prevailed the child's illness had little disruptive impact on the family unit'.

Tropauer made several other interesting points. First, the child's method of coping with cf exactly mirrored that of his parents. 'Patterns of deception and avoidance practised by the parents became the child's style of coping with the experience themselves.' Second, despite emotional conflicts and suffering 'most mothers retained the ability to perform their role' of supporting the child effectively. Indeed 'in some cases the closeness of the family bond was enhanced through sharing of grief or concern.'

This ability to transcend the infirmity was also noted in certain families by McCollum and Gibson (1971), who commented 'we have also noted instances in which parents have been able to maintain relationships with healthy children which are need fulfilling for the children, as well as deeply sustaining for the parents'. They conclude: 'perhaps this supports the premise that stress may result either in disorganisation or in deepening and consolidation of intrafamilial relationships.'

This conclusion prompts several fundamental queries. For example, how do some families flourish despite such heavy burdens? What enables one family to succeed whilst another fails? What are the factors which augment parental strength, and what are the factors which diminish it? None of these questions has ever been fully considered. Nor have previous studies attempted to assess the ways in which sick children manage to contain their natural anxieties and function effectively.

These therefore form the preoccupations of this present study. Its twin goals are: first, to assess the problems posed by cf for families who live in a welfare state, and are not additionally burdened by financial worries; second, to study and evaluate the ways in which parents and children are able to surmount the many anxieties and stresses which beset them.

The present study

To accomplish these aims it was clearly essential to contact a large, representative group of cf patients and their parents and discuss these topics with them. Because of the relative rarity of cf, it was felt that no one hospital could contribute a sufficient number of patients on its own. Similarly, it was felt that if one relied only on cf patients drawn from one hospital, there was a danger that the families seen might be economically or socially selected. It was, therefore, deemed essential to see families drawn from as wide an area as possible. Northern Ireland was chosen as a suitable area for research because it afforded access to families living in widely differing economic and social circumstances.[1] An attempt was therefore made, through the good auspices of local paediatricians, and the Cystic Fibrosis Research Trust, to contact all known cf families in Northern Ireland, and ultimately 54 families were traced. Only one complete family refused to participate in the study, though one mother and eight fathers were unavailable for interviewing when the work was actually commenced. In the event, 97 parents and 58 children were studied, drawn from 53 separate families (Table 1 gives details of family size and composition).

The parents

Parents were drawn from all social classes, though predictably the bulk fell into the Registrar General's category of skilled workers (Table 2 gives details of the differing socio-economic status of the fifty-three families, based on an assessment of the father's occupation). The average age of the mothers was thirty-three years, and the fathers thirty-six years. The mean family size was 4·0, but the group had sustained a high degree of child mortality prior to the study. Thirty-nine children had died previously, representing an overall mortality rate of 18 per cent (twenty-eight of these deaths were of diagnosed cf children). Understandably such loss had a profound effect on the psycho-social behaviour of parents and sick children.

[1] For comparison purposes a group of cf patients and their families was also studied in the east of Scotland by Dr W. M. McCrae and Mrs A. Cull. Reference to their findings is made, wherever applicable, throughout the text, and I would like to express my thanks to them for their collaboration.

Table 1 *Family size and composition*

Families studied	Cf children studied	Mothers interviewed	Fathers interviewed	Living sibs	Dead sibs
53 (Average no of children born 4·0)	58 (48 being the only cf child in family 10 having a cf sib)	52 (Average age 33 years, range 23-49)	45 (Average age 36 years, range 24-63)	112	39 (Mortality rate 18%)

Table 2 *Socio-economic classification of study families**

Class	No. of families
I	2
II	13
IIIM	15
IIINM	11
IV	1
V	9
Services	2
Total	53

*Based on the Registrar General's Classification of Occupations, 1970

Method of study—the parents

Each family member was visited in the privacy of his own home at a time which was most convenient to him. In this way meaningful communication was maximised and inconvenience minimised. On average each family was visited four times, the length of time taken varying enormously, the average being twenty hours. Mothers were normally seen first on two separate occasions, the first interview concentrating on the child's overall development and any practical difficulties caused by cf, and the second interview touching on the mother's own general wellbeing and any personal difficulties produced for her by the disease. Fathers were normally seen once, the interview focusing on their personal adjustment to the child's illness. In both interviews emphasis was placed on the parents' methods of overcoming the difficulties which they encountered. Interview schedules devised to elicit information regarding these topics were devised by me at the outset of the investigation.

The children

Table 3 gives details of the age and sex-distribution of the children concerned. The group was divided almost equally into pre-school and primary school-age children. Only two older cf children were to be found in Northern Ireland. Whilst there is a possibility that this lack of older children might result from misdiagnosis in earlier days (when techniques for identifying the disease were less accurate),

Table 3 *Age and sex distribution of the study children*

Study Children	Boys	Girls	Total
No.	33	25	58
Pre-school (up to 5 years)	15	12	27
Primary school (5-11 years)	16	13	29
Older than 11	2	—	2
Age range	7 mths-16·5 years	7 mths-10·6 years	
Average age	5 yrs 8 mths	5 yrs 3 mths	5·5 mths

these figures still bear witness to the high risk of early mortality associated with cf. Indeed, three study children—two boys and one girl—died during the period of the investigation, and full test results for them are not, therefore, available.

The clinical condition of the study children was assessed using the McCrae Scale, a rating scale which estimates the degree of chest involvement (Cull *et al.*, 1972). The children's health was thought to be best where, upon examination, the chest was clear and showed no signs of damage. Health became increasingly less good as bacteriological infection and damage to the lungs occurred. Using these criteria, 52 per cent of the fifty-eight Ulster children were thought to be in relatively good health, 17 per cent to be in moderate health, and 31 per cent to have chests which showed real evidence of damage and disease.[1]

Method of study—the children

During the course of the first interview with the mother, a very careful developmental history was taken. The mother was asked about every stage in the child's life, and invited to say how she and the child had coped with any difficulties which arose. Similarly, both father and mother were asked how they felt the child reacted to his illness and to the numerous stresses which it posed. In addition, for

[1] I am indebted to Dr John Dodge, Senior Lecturer, Dept of Child Health, The University Hospital of Wales, for assessing the study children on these physical parameters.

each pre-school child a Vineland Social Maturity Scale was completed, with the assistance of the mother.

Older children were interviewed separately in their own home at a time which was convenient to them. The interview began with a request for the child to draw first a man, then himself, and finally his family. This technique was used partly for its clinical value, and partly because it gave the child a relaxed half-hour in which to come to terms with the examiner. When these tasks were completed, each child was assessed using the Wechsler Intelligence Scale for Children, the Schonell Word Reading Test, the Schonell Spelling Test, and the Vernon Arithmetic Mathematics Test. Finally, an interview schedule devised by me dealing with the child's likes, dislikes, fears and aspirations was given, in addition to a standard Taylor Manifest Anxiety Scale. The session ended with each child making up six stories in response to pictures taken from the Thematic Apperception Test. In this way, it was possible to evaluate the child's intellectual potential, his academic attainment, and his personality functioning.

In addition, the class teacher of each school-age child was asked to assess his social functioning as it appeared in the classroom situation. For this purpose, a Bristol Social Adjustment Guide was used. In this respect, a comparison was made between subject children and a group of control children who were matched to the subject children in terms of intellectual potential, academic attainment, sex, age, socio-economic status, ordinal position in the family, and school attendance. Clearly, no comparison could be made in terms of comparability or chronicity of disease, though care was taken to match the severely handicapped subject children, who attended a special school for delicate children, with children equally handicapped by other disorders—asthma, heart trouble or chronic bronchitis.

In these different ways, every attempt was made to build up a complete picture of the study children and their parents.

2

Recognising preliminary symptoms and obtaining an adequate diagnosis

'That was the worst time of the lot, knowing something was wrong, and not knowing what.'

(Mother)

One of the first and most urgent problems facing parents of a chronically sick child is the problem of obtaining an adequate diagnosis. With some conditions this process, though painful, is relatively short-lived, for the child's initial symptoms are sufficiently severe to arrest immediate attention and recognition. Similarly, families with a previous history of chronic disease may be alerted early on to the possibility of recurrence, and their pre-diagnostic worries, though extreme, may also be relatively brief. Often, however, the search for an adequate diagnosis is a lengthy and painful one, involving parents in much unwarranted self-criticism. Preliminary symptoms may be ephemeral and confusing. The parents may question their own ability to detect these, and, if they meet with professional scepticism, they may become fundamentally confused and uncertain, doubting their own perceptions. Delays may result, endangering not only the child's health but the overall wellbeing of all family members. As a consequence, feelings of self-blame and guilt may occur, and hostility and mistrust may be engendered towards attendant medical personnel. All these observations were borne out by the experiences of the study families.

Children born with obvious disease symptoms

Three study children had mucus which was sufficiently tenacious to cause a bowel blockage within the first few days of life (meconium ileus). These children were diagnosed immediately, appropriate therapy was undertaken, and an adequate long-term treatment plan was evolved and explained to the parents. As a result, these parents, although severely shocked by the diagnosis (a factor discussed in greater detail in chapter 3), were none the less spared some of the painful uncertainty, which taxed parents of children with less obvious initial symptoms. This certainly reduced their overall level of distress.

Families with a previous history of chronic disease

Similarly 41 per cent of parents knew something of the disease prior to the birth of this affected child. Occasionally such knowledge sprang from the presence of another affected child within the home. More frequently it resulted from the previous death of a sick child. These parents were alerted to the possibility of recurrence long before the disease could actually be verified. Thus half these mothers felt certain, even whilst pregnant, that the baby they were carrying had the disease.

Mrs A. was a case in point. Her previous baby had died of cf at two months of age. A month later she accidentally conceived again. The loss of her previous baby had left her excessively depressed, and she became convinced that the expected baby would have the disease and also die. At five months she began to haemorrhage badly and had to rest in bed. As a result, she had to give up her job, thereby losing valuable earnings, a factor which added to her depression. Waiting—'the suspense was desperate'—she was totally demoralised, and the baby was induced two weeks early, weighing only 5 lb.

Not surprisingly, mothers like Mrs A. were continuously afraid throughout pregnancy, and consequently reported many symptoms indicative of considerable physical and emotional distress.[1]

---

[1] Interestingly, when considering the whole group (not solely those mothers who knew of cf prior to becoming pregnant), a surprisingly high incidence of physical and emotional distress during pregnancy was reported. Forty-nine per cent of mothers reported suffering from high blood pressure and toxaemia, and 83 per cent of mothers reported emotional distress or unsettling experiences during this pregnancy. Both these percentages are far in excess of the expected frequencies of such difficulties in Ulster, for example Dodge, 1972, cites a frequency of between 4 and 13 per cent for the different 'normal' control groups he used when studying the relationship of pregnancy stress to pyloric stenosis.

After the actual birth, 14 out of the 24 mothers with previous knowledge of the illness noticed confirmatory symptoms immediately and pressed urgently for diagnostic testing.

Thus Mrs C., who had lost two previous children, said: 'I definitely felt he would have it. He was born in hospital and yet they let him out three days later. He gained weight but I was sure myself he had it. He cried and wouldn't feed properly, so I took him in again at three weeks. They kept him in for two weeks, and then they told me he had a mild type of cf.'

Sometimes the unfortunate parents had to press for a diagnosis in the face of considerable medical scepticism. Thus Mrs S., who had already lost one son with cf, confided: 'I knew instinctively from birth he had it. I knew by his appearance that something was definitely wrong. I jumped to the conclusion it was the disease. I had a row with the gynaecologist because he wouldn't send him for a test. So I asked the GP to send him up to hospital. He said there was nothing wrong and not to be looking for trouble, it would show itself in time.'

Eventually Mrs S. effected a diagnosis by herself taking the baby to the hospital in which her other son died. There her anguish was perpetuated because of the difficulty of diagnosing the newborn in the absence of overwhelmingly obvious symptoms (such as those of meconium ileus). Her comments, typical of many, highlight the distress experienced by parents during the testing period. 'We kept ringing up. They said they were doing tests. It was a long time, two weeks at least. The suspense was desperate. At the end of that time they said they were treating him as if he had the disease.'

Occasionally parents who had lost previous children seemed reluctant to have the new baby tested, even though they sensed something was wrong. In several cases such mothers were eventually coaxed into allowing the baby to be tested by observant and conscientious health visitors. Thus, the only mother in the whole group who had not herself at any time sought medical help in effecting a diagnosis, commented: 'I had a notion something wasn't right, but you know what it is, you don't want to know for certain.' After some prevarication on her part, 'The nurse took him to the doctor, and he said she was fussing, but she insisted we went to a specialist and he did a sweat test and confirmed it.'

Despite these few mothers who were compelled to deny the severity of their child's condition for as long as possible, the diagnosis of this disease was made significantly earlier in the group with prior knowledge of the disease (Table 4).[1]

Table 4 *Average age at diagnosis of study children, related to symptomatology and disease history*

		No. of children	Average age of diagnosis (months)	Range in age of diagnosis (months)
Severe early symptoms		3	0	-
Slight symptoms	from families with previous history of disease	24	7	0-66
	from families with no previous history of disease	31	17	1-148

Families with no previous history of disease

Parents with no previous illness history to alert them to the severity of their child's condition, and no obvious initial symptoms, spent almost a year and a half on average in recognising their child's disease, and effecting an adequate diagnosis. During this time most were subjected to a bewildering array of symptoms, which tragically lent themselves to interpretation in many different ways. As one father tersely commented, 'every alternative explanation . . . was so reasonable'. The apparent reasonableness of alternative explanations not only delayed the parents' initial search for medical help, but also delayed the obtaining of an accurate diagnosis once such help was requested. Thus many parents experienced a long-drawn-out pre-diagnostic saga of self-doubts, eventual medical interviews, reasonable alternative explanations, ineffective treatments, more self-doubts, despair, more medical interviews and so on. This saga undoubtedly potentiated their eventual sense of shock and despair in hearing the diagnosis. Cases such as the following were not uncommon:

[1] The median age of diagnosis of the children with slight symptoms was five months. A χ^2 test was used to assess the difference between the numbers of children above or below the median in families with differing disease histories. $\chi^2 = 6.76$ df $= 1$ p < 0.01.

'When he was born he weighed 7lb. 4oz., and in hospital he kept bringing up his bottles, and they said it was mucus in the stomach, and when I brought him back he kept bringing up bottles and his motions had an awful smell, and he kept losing weight. At five months he was only 13lb. and my family doctor kept coming and he said it was just sinus—but each bottle he took came straight up and his motions ran all over the pram.'

Another mother described her baby's pre-diagnostic difficulties:

'Well, he developed a cold and I took him to our GP and he said he'd got a bad bout of flu and gave him penicillin and said this would clear him up, and I waited a week and he started to puff and wheeze and he was no better and I took him back, and the doctor said he'd got an infection and I took him into hospital but the wheeze didn't clear, though they said it would—just to take him home. But the wheezing went on, and he couldn't breathe and then they took him in in March and kept him in until June. They did tests. They thought it was asthma, then bronchitis, then cf. Then they took him to London for a second opinion. I never had him. I didn't know I had a baby.'

Reassessing methods of child-rearing

The problem of accurately identifying early symptoms was compounded by the fact that many of them seemed nothing more than persistent and exaggerated forms of more common, babyhood complaints. For example, 69 per cent of babies had presented feeding difficulties during the first three months of life. Over 30 per cent continued to have feeding problems up to and beyond the first year. Not unexpectedly—in view of the initial preponderance of pregnancy stress—these babies tended to be sick or refuse nourishment. Only a few presented the classic cf symptom of voracious appetite. Fifty-nine per cent of babies failed to gain weight satisfactorily. In many cases parents felt that these difficulties were due to their own mismanagement of the baby's care, and such feelings were accentuated by the gratuitous comments of neighbours and family. Often mothers felt compelled to change their basic child-rearing methods several times before they accepted that the baby's difficulties were not of their own making. Such experiences diminished their natural self-confidence and understandably distressed them; for example, 80 per cent of mothers whose babies were failing to thrive said they had experienced considerable emotional distress because of this. One such mother said, 'From a couple of weeks old I knew something was wrong. That was the worst time of the lot, knowing something was wrong and not knowing what.'

Seeking a diagnosis

Understandably, most parents faced with such distressing early difficulties sought the help of their medical advisers. In 11 cases (including the 3 with meconium ileus) the parents went immediately to a paediatrician. In the remaining 47 cases the parents went first to a GP and eventually through him to a paediatrician. Whilst in 16 cases diagnosis was effected with remarkable speed after this initial interview, in 73 per cent of cases diagnosis was delayed. Twenty-three per cent of mothers were told they were 'fussy', 'imagining things', or 'nuts'. Forty per cent of mothers were initially given an incorrect diagnosis. Such preliminary diagnoses ranged from 'he's on the wrong food', 'he's got bronchitis', 'it's a baby thing and he'll outgrow it', to heart or coeliac disease. Eight per cent of mothers were told that the doctor did not know what was wrong, and one mother had her daughter placed on treatment without being told what it was for. Unsuspectingly, she conceived a second baby with the disease who died shortly after birth, when finally the first child's condition was explained to her.

Several observations emerge from a careful assessment of the statements parents made concerning their search for an adequate diagnosis.

1 Medical scepticism   Diagnosis was most usually made in the face of much medical scepticism and required considerable parental energy to effect; for example, the professional mother of a firstborn girl said:

> 'I noticed from ten days old she was odd, and my fears increased over the next months, and our health visitor and district nurse both thought she was not doing well. They weighed her and thought she was small, and I knew she hadn't put on weight and wasn't feeding well, and then I went to the local baby clinic at six weeks and told them she was not eating well, and having

diarrhoea and rashes, but they wouldn't take me seriously and they said "there are some small babies and some big babies". Then I went to stay with my husband's parents in another town and we went to the baby clinic there—but again they didn't take me seriously. Then I went to our family doctor and said I didn't think she was thriving well, and he couldn't see anything wrong, and so at three months I went to another GP who immediately knew she was unwell, and said to go to a paediatrician, and so we went back to our GP and demanded to see a paediatrician.'

Another mother, the wife of a semi-skilled worker, who had lost one previous child and did not accomplish the diagnosis of the second child until she was fifteen months old, said:

'She had terrible diarrhoea from the beginning. If you gave her a bottle, it squirted out. Every time you looked at her it squirted out. I'll never forget her first winter—not putting on weight. Always a round fat face, but so thin. I took her to our doctor but he had no idea. He said I was nuts, there was nothing wrong with her. He kept finding nothing wrong at all. Everybody, even my own mother was saying there was nothing wrong with her, I felt if I didn't find out something was wrong with her, I would know I was nuts.'

General—and especially medical—scepticism of this sort undermined the parents' self-confidence, and their faith in their own powers of perception. Not surprisingly, therefore, parents whose early forebodings were dismissed as nonsense or imagination were subsequently more resentful of medical personnel than those who were told that the doctor didn't know what was wrong, or who were first given an incorrect diagnosis. In both these latter situations the parents at least had their initial misgivings confirmed, and they were more willing to forgive subsequent delays in ascertaining the exact nature of the disease. Similarly, once the doctor had in some way acknowledged the reality of the child's illness state, parents felt more secure in pursuing the matter to its logical conclusion. By contrast, those who had their early misgivings dismissed lightly were made more insecure and self-critical as parents, often not only to the detriment of the infant-parent relationship, but also to the vigour with which they sought further medical help.

These comments were certainly borne out by the experiences of many parents. For example, one mother who had had her first child die of the disease, did not accomplish the diagnosis of the second until she was over four years of age. She had early been put off by being told that she was 'fussing unduly'. She said, 'I just tried, but I thought . . . other people said I was fussing a bit. I wasn't sure if I was or if she was unwell. I just knew there was something wrong.'

2 *Parental insecurity exacerbated by scepticism*   Parents who particularly doubted their own instinctive nurturant abilities, for example, very young parents, or parents of first-born children, seemed to be most distressed by medical scepticism. Thus a teenage mother said:

'I went to the baby clinic every week. She would gain 1lb. one week, and lose it the next. They said I was fussing unnecessarily. They said there were skinny and fat babies, and I was fussing too much. I went to a doctor and he gave me some stuff and he said, "You're a young mother, are you sure you won't put it in her ear instead of her mouth." It made me feel a fool.'

Another mother, previously a nurse, commented: 'I was a nurse before and I should have insisted on his doing something earlier—but I thought perhaps I was a nervous mother and imagining things. You had to trust him.'

The teenage mother of a first-born child added:

'I had to keep feeding him every two hours, night and day. I thought I was going to the mad house. He never slept. He was always being sick. I kept going to our family doctor, and in the end he was getting browned off, and he said to my mother—she used to go with me—"Talk a bit of sense into the girl, get her to stop annoying me!" I knew he wasn't right—but with a first child you don't realise so much.'

Not surprisingly such episodes diminished the parents' attempts to obtain an adequate diagnosis, increased their sense of frustration, and were conducive to considerable subsequent hostility.

3 *The usefulness of objective support*   Parents who were well supported, either by their immediate family, or by a sensitive health visitor, or district nurse, seemed to fare best. To illustrate this, 81

per cent of mothers had been visited in the baby's early days by a health visitor, and 53 per cent said they found these visits helpful. Generally this was because the health visitor provided moral support, listening to the mother, and taking her misgivings seriously. In several instances it was the health visitor who was directly responsible for effecting the diagnosis by confirming the mother's suspicions regarding the ailing infant, upholding her in her dialogue with medical personnel, and pressing for adequate testing of the sick child.

4 The relationship of parental social class to speed of child's diagnosis Parents who found it hard to communicate adequately with their doctor, or who doubted their own ability to perceive subtle changes in their child's physical state were often deflected from their diagnostic quest by medical scepticism. Consequently, it was the more intelligent, more articulate, and more determined parents who most speedily effected diagnosis. Confirming this point, Table 5 gives details of the age at diagnosis of infants born to parents of differing socio-economic classes. Because of the size of the sample, three main groupings were used, combined classes I and II, III M and III NM, and IV and V (based on parental occupations as assessed by the Registrar General's Classification of Occupations, 1970).[1]

Table 5 indicates that parents in the professional and managerial classes (I and II) effect a diagnosis more speedily than either skilled parents (III M and III NM) or semi- and unskilled parents (IV and V), and this observation held true whether the family had any previous history of disease to guide them, or whether they were merely struggling in the dark.

Several factors may account for the relationship between speed of diagnosis and socio-economic class of parent. First, communication may be better between doctors and professional and managerial parents, simply because the latter are better able to comprehend and use medical terminology. They can then deploy this on their child's behalf, arresting more immediate attention. Second, the more intelligent parents may find it easier to obtain confirmation of their suspicions from textbooks and paediatric manuals. This not only

[1] Two service families were excluded from analysis because parental occupation placed them in a separate socio-economic category, the numbers of which were insufficient for individual analysis.

Table 5 *Age at diagnosis of children born in differing socio-economic groups* [1]

Children	Age	I and II	IIIM and IIINM	IV and V
Families with no previous disease history	Mean age at diagnosis (months)	8·4	15·0	36·3
	Range (months)	3-24	1-54	3-148
	No.	7	16	6
Families with previous knowledge of disease	Mean age at diagnosis (months)	2·1	9·2	11·0
	Range (months)	0-6	0-66	0-30
	No.	8	10	6

obviates their own initial uncertainty, making for greater—rather than less—efforts in effecting a diagnosis, but also information gleaned in this way provides ammunition when pressing for the child's needs to be taken seriously. Third, professional and managerial parents may be more likely than skilled or semi-skilled parents to have friends with medical or paramedical skills upon whom they can call for confirmatory assistance. They are therefore less likely to be solely reliant on the single assessment of their GP or baby clinic doctor.

To illustrate this point, one university-trained mother kept a diary of her infant's symptoms from two weeks of age. She was initially alerted to the possibility of a problem because of the colour of the baby's stools. She then 'had a succession of midwives, doctors and nurse friends looking at him'. On the basis of their comments she continued to press her GP to have the baby tested by a paediatrician. This was effected within two months. Then, as the father put it:

'At first we thought he had "malabsorption" and we looked up "malabsorption" and found "cystic fibrosis", and then we

[1] This table excludes the meconium ileus children, who were all diagnosed within a few days.

looked up "cystic fibrosis" and we also read an article on coeliac disease, and we knew a sweat test was for cystic fibrosis and then we 'phoned a doctor friend who knew a fair bit.'

Not only did such social contacts, and access to knowledge speed up diagnosis, but they generally facilitated the parents' overall comprehension of the illness once the diagnosis was established (a factor considered in greater detail in chapter 4). For example, in terms of the parents' comprehension of the long-term genetic risks attached to this illness, fathers who showed the best understanding had left school on average at 16·1 years, fathers who showed moderate or poor understanding had left school at 14·8 years,*[1] and fathers with no understanding of genetic risks had left school at 14·3 years.[2]

5 *Hostility engendered in parents towards medical advisers* As might be expected, difficulties encountered in effecting the diagnosis stimulated feelings of hostility in parents towards their medical advisers. Comments such as these were not uncommon: 'I did feel angry towards him because the child didn't get the proper treatment at first.' 'I felt very hostile. I asked my husband, was there any legal procedure I could take against him.' In all, 39 per cent of mothers blamed their medical advisers for not recognising the disease straight away, and several mothers either changed their GPs or sought legal advice with a view to prosecution. Twenty-eight per cent of mothers added that these experiences had radically altered their attitude to the medical profession, generally for the worse. Feelings of blame thus engendered seemed to bear little relationship to the objective length of delay encountered in effecting the diagnosis; rather they seemed more closely related to the parents' own subjective sense of loss because of delay. This was clearly illustrated by the comments of parents relating to the possible damage to their child which might have resulted. A father commented: 'Our doctor's delay could have killed her, had she had a serious infection. All the time she was getting weaker, and her symptoms were stronger.' A mother commented: 'If she had been detected earlier she would have

---

* Differences between groups were assessed statistically and found to be significantly different, using the t test.

[1] $t = 2·07$, df = 27, $p < 0·05$.

[2] $t = 2·14$, df = 15, $p < 0·05$.

had less lung damage and not pneumonia—which is the worst thing that could have happened to her.'

Two other factors potentiated hostility; first, not having been taken seriously by the doctor: 'The one thing that did annoy me was that they wouldn't believe me when I was so sure something was wrong'; and, second, the knowledge that the doctor already had experience with this condition and should have been able to detect it: 'He had another child on his panel with cf. I wouldn't have expected him to recognise cf if he hadn't another child with it.' This particularly applied to those twenty-four sets of parents who had already lost previous children. When they experienced delay in effecting diagnosis, they were especially bitter: 'They should have kept a better watch on it after that.'

Conversely, feelings of anger abated when parents realised the rarity of cf: 'Our doctor came up and apologised and said he'd never treated a case before. We couldn't expect him to recognise something he hadn't seen before.' 'We blamed him at the time but after we read the literature we realised he would only see one of these children once in his time.' In addition, where the doctor made efforts—as was usually the case—to be attentive, seemed concerned, expressed regret, or visited regularly he was forgiven. Also, some parents were swift to appreciate the ill-advisability of quarrelling, or taking lasting umbrage against someone upon whom they were so obviously dependent. A mother summarised such feelings thus: 'Sometimes it makes me very bitter, but I can't just turn round and blame the doctor. I still feel I need him a lot and I can't say outright.'

Generally, parents felt their experiences had made them more wary of unquestioningly accepting medical advice, and they blamed themselves as much as the doctor for previously unreasonable expectations in this respect. As one mother said: 'I now know they don't know everything. I used to think that they did. People are in awe of doctors. You know they've studied and looked into things and you think they know everything—and then you realise they don't. They're just people.'

Often such realisations increased the parents' own natural sense of authority and self-confidence, repairing some of the damage done by the initially sceptical environment. For example, 'We feel now we can tell the doctors a lot, because the doctors are not with them all the time, and working with a child you can find out a lot.' 'Since then we press things, we don't let them slide.' 'I feel I can talk better to him now. We can find out together what is wrong, rather than him telling me.'

As a result of these initial difficulties, very few families ultimately placed much reliance on their family doctor, either as a source of information concerning the disease (discussed in greater detail in chapter 4) or as a source of help regarding treatment difficulties (dealt with in chapter 6). Instead, parents turned increasingly to paediatricians as a source of guidance. Thus, whilst 69 per cent of mothers and 39 per cent of fathers thought the paediatrician was of very much or moderate help to them in understanding the disease, only 22 per cent of mothers and 13 per cent of fathers deemed their GP of equal value.

6 Parental self-blame and recrimination A very small percentage of parents blamed themselves for not seeking medical help for their child sooner. Generally, as with blame directed towards medical personnel, such feelings seemed less related to the objective length of delay, but were more closely related to the parents' fears regarding possible resultant damage. For example, one mother said: 'I felt I wasn't quick enough—one of her lungs has a great scar—it's bad for her age.'

Most parents fortunately avoided such guilty feelings by assuming a fatalistic approach. 'It was just one of those things. I suppose had she died it would have been different. I would have been angry.' 'I don't blame anyone. None of us could really tell, and they can't prevent it anyway.'

Probably the overall feeling was not so much one of self-blame but of regret, a wistful lingering sense of 'if only'.

3

Learning the diagnosis

'I can't recall what we were told on that occasion. An awful lot
of what he said I lost. I'd already begun to look out of the
window. The feeling I had the roof was coming in around us.
When you're listening to that you're miles away—it isn't
happening—you're detached.'

(*Father*)

Most parents experience a very real need to care for and protect their
children throughout the course of their development. The diagnosis
of a chronic disease threatens the fulfilment of this need and as such
it represents a massive attack on the integrity and wellbeing of most
parents. Not surprisingly, therefore, most respond to the stress with
an initial sense of shock or stunning, and when this wears off and
reality impinges, many mobilise defence mechanisms to ward off the
implications of this threat. The reality of the illness symptoms may
be denied, the physician's competence questioned, or parents may
search for alternative opinions. When all these gambits fail, parents
may respond by becoming increasingly dispirited, lacking in self-
esteem, and mourning for the well child whom they have lost.

All these behaviours have been noted in the responses of parents
facing up to the diagnosis of a malignant disease (Burton, 1971).
Similarly, the ninety-seven parents of children with cf demonstrated
that this pattern of defence is not specific to malignancy, but
constant, occurring whenever any such threat to the stability of the
family unit is made.

Before one can understand how parents respond to diagnosis it is essential to discover how the news was broken. Because of the chronic and serious nature of cf I presumed that both parents would automatically be together when the doctor imparted the facts, and consequently that both parents would be better able to support one another. Sadly, this assumption was ill-founded. Whilst all of the 52 mothers interviewed had been present at diagnosis, only 37 per cent of fathers (20 out of a potential 53) accompanied their wives on this occasion. Understandably this lack of togetherness potentiated maternal distress, and diminished the parents' overall understanding of the disease.

Several reasons were advanced to account for the father's absence. Occasionally pressing work commitments made absence unavoidable, but more often it occurred simply because no one had alerted the parents in advance concerning the severity of the situation. As a consequence, the mother unsuspectingly turned up alone—often on the day of discharge—bringing the child's clothes and expecting to take him home. Few anticipated anything more than a routine interview with the paediatrician concerned.

In such circumstances it was only the most anxious, determined or subjectively alerted fathers who seized this opportunity to assess their child's condition with his doctor—in short, the very parents who had pushed most strenuously for early diagnosis. Not surprisingly, therefore, the highest proportion of fathers present at diagnosis came from the ranks of the managerial and professional classes (Table 6 gives details of the proportion of fathers (excluding

Table 6 *Fathers present at diagnosis according to socio-economic class*

	I and II	*III M and III NM*	*IV and V*
Fathers present (%)	64	30	18
No.	15	26	10

Service personnel) present according to socio-economic class). Similarly, proportionately more skilled fathers were present when compared with semi- or unskilled fathers. One is forced to conclude that, at least in part, the greater the intelligence, and natural authority of the parent concerned, the more likely he is to be subjectively aware of the significance of his child's early symptoms, and—whether or not he is objectively alerted—the more enthusiastically he will pursue diagnosis.

Other possible explanations for the greater preponderance of the higher socio-economic classes at diagnosis might include: (1) a greater flexibility of role among such parents, which allowed for accompanying wives to hospital on such occasions; (2) a greater preparedness to communicate with medical authorities; (3) a greater enthusiasm on the doctor's part to meet such parents. All of these suppositions were borne out by the comments of parents involved. For example, an unskilled father said: 'I've never met the doctor. He's never wanted to see me. My wife has taken all to do with him, and has been very good. I'm very fortunate. It's taken the burden off my shoulders.'

Another unskilled father from a rural area added: 'No doctors have ever talked to me. Any talking would be with the mammy.' This particular father defined his paternal role as 'providing for them until fit to provide for themselves—that's a father's job, and the mother's is to mind them'.

For this father, the acts of going to learn the diagnosis and removing the child from hospital on the day of discharge were clearly viewed as essential parts of 'minding' the child, viz. woman's work.

Understanding the diagnosis

Understandably, those fathers who were not present when the diagnosis was imparted could not be expected to have as complete a comprehension of the basic facts relating to the disease as their wives, no matter how carefully the latter might relay the news. It was not therefore surprising to discover that as a group fathers were generally less well informed at the outset concerning the illness. Table 7 illustrates this point. Parents were asked whether three basic facts relating to their child's disease had been imparted to them at the time of diagnosis. The majority of mothers said they had been told at least some of these facts, whereas the majority of fathers said they had not.

Table 7 *Parents who said basic information was available to them at the time of diagnosis*

	Mothers	Fathers
The disease was chronic, requiring constant treatment (%)	75	57
The disease was inherited (%)	74	30
The disease could get worse in the future (%)	55	33
No.	52	45

Parents were allotted a score in terms of the number of basic facts they received at diagnosis and were later able to recollect. Table 8 gives details of the average scores obtained by both sexes, according to social class.

Mothers from all socio-economic groupings resemble each other closely in terms of the amount of information they received and were able to recollect. Fathers differed however, those from the higher socio-economic classes absorbing and retaining most. This relationship held true whether or not the father was present at diagnosis, though the best parental comprehension was found amongst those professional and managerial fathers who attended the diagnostic interview.

Two factors may account for this apparent relationship between social class and parental understanding of illness at diagnosis. First,

Table 8 *Average factual score obtained by parents for information imparted at diagnosis, according to sex and social class*

	I and II	III M and III NM	IV and V
Mothers	2·0	2·2	2·0
All fathers	1·3	1·1	0·75
Fathers present at diagnosis only	1·8	1·1	0·0

the more able fathers were possibly better equipped to grasp and remember the complex concepts involved, and also to understand the doctor's attempts at communicating these. However, too much reliance on this proposition is not possible because no similar differences in understanding according to social class were observed amongst the wives. More probably, the relationship stems from role expectations. While most mothers see their role as that of caring for their child, and are therefore eager to grasp relevant information, fathers generally, and especially those in the lower socio-economic classes, view such matters as more properly the concern of their wives, and are therefore less prepared to absorb facts relating to the illness.

However, it is obvious from a scrutiny of Tables 7 and 8 that whatever the social class of the parents concerned, many felt they were deprived at the outset of some basic facts regarding the disease. The chronic nature of the illness, and the need for treatment, seemed more generally appreciated by both sexes than other more complex and possibly more frightening facts, such as the inherited nature of the disease, and the long-term possibility of a poor prognosis. In part this could be due to the fact that some clinicians may deliberately phase the delivery of such information, retaining certain less threatening and possibly less essential details until later interviews, when parents could better be expected to cope with them. In part also these disparities in comprehension may be due to an instinctive warding off of the more distressing details.

The parents' sense of shock at diagnosis

It is now well recognised that the diagnosis of chronic and possibly fatal illness in a child represents a massive threat to the integrity and personal stability of most parents. As such the news resembles some grievous personal accident, and is responded to with a sense of shock or stunning. In such a state many parents cannot believe the diagnosis. Occasionally, they do not even hear it. This point was amply borne out in my conversations with these parents. For example, one skilled father who was present commented:

'I can't recall what we were told on that occasion. An awful lot of what he said I lost. I'd already begun to look out of the window. The feeling I had the roof was coming in around us.

When you're listening to that you're miles away—it isn't happening—you're detached.'

A mother added:

'I just felt stunned. I couldn't take it in. Maybe it wasn't explained fully enough then—even the name didn't register. I didn't know what it was. If we'd been brought back after the initial shock it would have been better . . . when you hear these things your mind goes in a whirl.'

Another mother confided: 'I didn't even know what it was. I thought it was multiple sclerosis. I couldn't remember what it was she had. I kept crying, but I didn't know. The CF Trust Secretary had to come up and explain it to me.'

Being alone at such a time intensified the agony of many mothers. For example, one young mother said:

'I couldn't even come home when she told me. I was very shattered. I couldn't even drive home. I had to 'phone my sister for help. . . . I couldn't even tell my husband what was wrong. I could only see death. Just death. I couldn't even see my other little boy. When he came up to me I couldn't touch him. He got on my nerves a lot, and I just cried for three days.'

Another mother described her feelings thus:

'I walked home from the hospital. There was snow on the ground. I just wanted to walk and walk. It was all a blank and life stood still. I couldn't go on a bus for fear of crying . . . all that kept running through my head was "an incurable disease" —as if the wheels of the bus kept saying it. She would never get over it.'

This initial sense of shock could last for many days, as witnessed by the following observation:

'When I got the baby home I was still numb. I used to walk around in a daze and people said I was very stuck up. I used to just sit listlessly for hours, and I thought I'd go mad he cried so much and needed so much attention.'

Similarly on occasions shock could be delayed until after the child's immediate safety was assured. Thus one mother observed:

'It didn't hit us at once . . . it didn't seem to penetrate. He was so poorly and the doctors didn't give him much chance. I just accepted it. The doctors said he wouldn't last long. Then he started to pull round and got better and it was sort of delayed action, I was shocked later.'

Parental loss of esteem, and self-criticism following diagnosis

Whilst initially parents may be too shocked to appreciate the reality of what they are told, gradually the significance of the diagnosis cannot be avoided. Profound feelings of depression, lowered self-esteem and worthlessness ensue. The parents blame themselves for the child's condition, and critically review their attitudes and behaviour towards him. Such self-criticism stems either from the parents' sense of guilt in failing adequately to protect their child from trauma, or from their attempt to understand and come to terms with the event. Most parents in our society have been reared to believe that conformity and good behaviour will be rewarded, and where their child is diagnosed as having a chronic disorder they find themselves in a situation in which they are both singled out and punished. In terms of the rules by which they have previously lived, this seems only possible as a result of some failure on their own part, and they therefore seek to establish this 'fact', thereby making sense of the event, and supporting their previous ideology. Conversely, where parents come to believe that the child's illness was a chance event or 'a trick of fate', they frequently question both the meaning of life, and ultimately their own sanity.

All these observations were borne out by the comments of the parents themselves; for example one mother said: 'I used to feel, why has it got to happen to me with just one. There are hordes of children who are not looked after, not wanted.'

Another mother of a first baby said: 'I felt it was very unfair. I kept asking , "what did I ever do for this?", but my mother said it had nothing to do with me.'

The mother of a two-year-old boy confided: 'I felt this had happened because I had insisted on bringing him to the doctor. I blamed myself more than them.' Another mother added: 'I thought there must be something seriously wrong with my husband and myself—like the plague—and we'd passed it on to her. I couldn't understand it.'

Often such feelings were extremely complex, producing substantial changes in wider relationships; for example, one mother who had lost two previous children said:

'I kept asking why was it happening to me. Some people have seven, and they're all healthy, and I've had five and three have had this disease, and I had a grudge against people. At the beginning I didn't like to see wee babies or watch them on TV, even my other boys. There was a blankness . . . they didn't seem to be mine at all.'

Occasionally, such feelings were extended even to the sick child. A mother who experienced such feelings told me: 'I find it harder to love her . . . in case I lose her. . . . I'm scared of getting too close to her. I don't think I've drawn away, but our relationship just hasn't developed. I could be closer to her.'

Denial of diagnosis

Understandably, such thoughts and feelings only accentuated the parents' existent emotional turmoil, and almost invariably were countered by defence mechanisms aimed at reducing the emotional pain, or affording the individual sufferer some minimal control over his feelings. Denial of diagnosis was probably the most widespread of these defence mechanisms, with parents actively questioning the implications of what they were told. The following comments were typical: 'I thought he might be wrong, and there was nothing wrong with the child at all.' 'I felt it wasn't it. She hasn't got it at all, that she couldn't have it.' A father added: 'I can't really describe how I felt about it at the time. It's sort of a thing you don't think about . . . you push it more into the back of your mind and don't think of it.'

Whilst such denial predominated immediately following diagnosis, it was very long-lasting and frequently took much time to abate. At the time of the survey—which was on average four and a half years after the child's diagnosis—26 per cent of mothers and 39 per cent of fathers still doubted the implications of what they had been told. Denial tended to escalate when the child was well, and inevitably diminished with any exacerbation of serious symptoms.

People cannot experience such a gamut of emotions without significant side-effects. In the context of their understanding of the illness, perhaps the most crucial of these is a diminution in their ability to comprehend what is said. Not only do they actively not want to know, but also they experience a paralysis of thought processes which renders impossible comprehension of anything but the simplest, clearest information.

Thus, whilst 53 per cent of the mothers and 17 out of the 20 fathers, who were present at diagnosis, thought the doctor had been tactful and kindly in his method of imparting the news—and several of those who found him brusque felt this was more directly attributable to their own sense of shock rather than his manner—many parents spontaneously commented that they could not understand what had been said. The following comments were typical: 'They talk in big words and half the time you can't understand.' 'He came out with a lot of big words—medical words. I wouldn't have understood.'

Occasionally such lack of understanding seemed more directly attributable to medical abstruseness, rather than to the parents' denial, and, as a consequence, six mothers said that they found it so hard to understand the information they were given that they completely failed to grasp the severity of the situation. As a result, they experienced little emotional disturbance. Thus, one mother confided: 'It didn't register properly at first for we'd never heard of it before. The consultant said what he'd got and how it had to be treated—but it didn't really register.' Another added: 'I didn't appreciate how serious it was. I knew nothing of it. They just said she'd got cf and that was all—unless he thought I already knew, and whenever I came home I tried to remember to tell my husband.'

Obviously such comments argue both for a studied simplicity of verbal presentation, and also for the giving of basic information in written form so that parents can take it home and study it when they are calmer.

The need for phasing the delivery of basic illness information

A further possibility in terms of maximising comprehension is for the physician to arrange for the parents to visit him on several different occasions following the diagnosis of a chronic disease. In this way, he can gently impart all the necessary facts at a speed which keeps pace with the parents' own natural adjustment to the threatening situation.

Most parents would have been grateful for the provision of such facilities. Then they could have gradually absorbed, reaffirmed and clarified the complex information they were given. One typical father commented: 'There were lots of questions that weren't asked, for we were trying to absorb what he was telling us. . . . It is some time before your mind settles down to accepting the fact, and then you want to enquire more.'

A teenage mother found her own mother's presence at diagnosis of immense value in this respect. 'Only for my mother that night I would have been really lost. She threw questions at him which I couldn't have thrown.'

In view of this obvious need for phasing the delivery of the diagnostic information, it was sad to find that such facilities were available in only 43 per cent of cases. This was indeed a deprivation, for in those cases where the doctor was available for consultation on subsequent occasions over 70 per cent of parents availed themselves of the opportunity and returned to discuss the child's illness at a less traumatic time.

Relationship of parental shock to expectation and preparedness

Where parents believed, prior to diagnosis, that their child had only some minimal defect, their sense of shock seemed most profound. Thus whilst just over half of all the mothers interviewed reported feelings of shock at being given the news, all of the mothers with no previous knowledge of cf, and no real idea that the child was seriously unwell, experienced severe shock.

The converse was also true. Where parents had been led to believe that the child's life was in jeopardy, they accepted the diagnosis of chronic disease more easily. Thus one father commented:

'I think we were expecting it and the fact he had had a blood transfusion. We thought of leukaemia, and he was always very pale, and we were almost expecting him not to survive, and when we got the diagnosis, and were told of children of seven with cf who were living—that was a relief.'

The mother of a two-year-old girl commented: 'When the doctor told me I thought she was going to die, and each time I went she seemed worse. It was better really for if I'd been expecting her to live it would have been worse.' Another mother added: 'I think I had prepared myself for it before. I am a bit of a pessimist and my husband is an optimist—and it was worse for him. I felt relief at being told.'

Perhaps because of some innate appreciation of the value of preparation for such news, half the parents interviewed said how grateful they would have been for some earlier indication that things were seriously amiss. One such father commented: 'I prefer to be kept in the picture as much as possible, and to be told what type of investigation they're following and what's happening, because I think being kept in the dark makes you more worried.' A mother added: 'If only they had given us some enlightenment that things weren't as they should have been, it wouldn't have come as such a shock. They never even told us about the tests.'

This latter point seemed a real thorn in the flesh of many parents, possibly because it could be used as a focus for the expression of pent-up hostilities engendered by the appalling frustration of the situation.

Thus a father remembered entering the ward, and seeing his daughter having a blood transfusion. He was anguished by 'the shock of not knowing what it was for. The nurse there didn't know why.' A mother observed:

> 'I don't think it's right to start testing without telling us what for. They used to do this in hospital, with notices on the door and tubes up his nose, and liquid going in, and it frightened me, and shocked me. They could have warned me. They used to ask me to save nappies, but they never explained why.'

A professional father commented bitterly: 'They never levelled with us once.'

The need for honesty at diagnosis

The enormous importance of this latter point was emphasised by the general agreement found amongst parents concerning the need for complete honesty on the physician's part once he actually knew what was wrong. Comments such as: 'I was glad she told me the truth at the time,' and 'We told him frankly we would prefer to hear all about it,' were common.

Often this attitude was justified because 'Blunt or not you want the truth . . . that's the only way you're going to learn to accept it,' or 'What you know you can face. What you don't know you can't face.'

By being told everything honestly at the outset, parents felt they were saved extra unnecessary worry and suspense.

The relationship of parental shock to age of child at diagnosis

To some extent, this last conclusion may be further substantiated by the fact that the longer the child's pre-diagnostic difficulties continued, the more likely was his mother to report severe shock on being given the news. Thus the mean age at diagnosis of the infants of thirty-four mothers who reported shock was 14·8 months (range = 0-14 years), compared with a mean age at diagnosis of 8·5 months (range = 0-3 years) of children of mothers who did not feel shocked at learning the news.

This apparent relationship between age of child at diagnosis and parental shock may derive in two ways. First, mothers of infants may be more prepared for their loss than mothers of older children; witness the not uncommon first question to the midwife: 'Is he all right?' Second, the older the child, the more his parents may be attached to him. Certainly many parents emphasised this latter point in their comments. Thus a father said: 'If anything had happened to him then, it wouldn't have hit me so much as now, after three years. At a couple of months you haven't the same attachment.' A mother said: 'We were prepared to lose her at the start, but as time goes on, it gets harder.'

Maternal fears for the child following diagnosis

Mothers were asked about their worries concerning the child following diagnosis. Sixty-three per cent said they were mainly concerned with the child's survival, and only secondarily with how they would themselves cope. For example, one mother confided: 'I worried in terms of the future—could she live? I would do anything in my power to keep her alive—just as long as she's living—even if I had to push her around in a wheelchair for the rest of her life.' Another mother said: 'I kept thinking about the future. I looked at all her baby clothes and thought she would never wear them—we'd never have her.'

Such fears could reach phobic proportions; for example, one mother said she was unable to enter her daughter's bedroom in the morning, after being told. She commented: 'I make my husband go in and look at her first. I have a terrible dread I might see her lying there dead.'

Such fears could be very persistent, continuing even though the child, on necessary treatment, began to thrive. The mother of a six-year-old girl, who was progressing very satisfactorily, commented: 'You say you don't worry but you do. If she even coughs in the night I wonder is this the last night I'm going to have her. I worry so much about her. I have such fear.'

Mothers with differing illness histories and from all social classes had such fears. In addition, 31 per cent of mothers were worried about how they would care for the child, or cope with the illness symptoms or necessary treatment regime. Worries concerning care seemed related both to social class and illness history. Thus, only 20 per cent of the professional and middle class mothers expressed such concern, as against 45 per cent of class III mothers and 42 per cent of mothers from classes IV and V. Similarly, mothers with previous knowledge of the disease expressed twice as many fears relating to caring for the child, compared with mothers who were meeting the disease for the first time. Probably this relationship occurs because mothers with previous knowledge of the illness are only too well aware of the considerable burden which is placed upon them by the required treatment regime.

Comments such as the following were often heard:

'He was four months old when we got him out of hospital. He weighed nine pounds. I was terrified about his immediate care. He looked like a Biafran. I was dreadful afraid to take him home. I nearly had a heart attack when I saw what he looked like.'

'My first reaction was for myself. Would I be able to cope with it? I was very worried for myself. Afraid I wouldn't be able to look after him properly myself. I was afraid to have him in the house.'

Understandably, the fears and responsibilities attendant on the child's diagnosis had repercussions on the general wellbeing of the parents. As a consequence, 87 per cent of mothers and 60 per cent of fathers reported experiencing one or more physically distressing symptom which they attributed solely to worry over their child's condition. The most common symptom was depression, with 44 per cent of mothers and 33 per cent of fathers experiencing it. Other difficulties were nervousness, sleep difficulties, and disorders of appetite. Usually such physical sequelae emerged unexpectedly, though in a few instances parents admitted that these health problems had been in existence prior to the affected child's birth, and were merely exacerbated by his diagnosis.

To some extent, such symptoms expressed a syndrome of anticipatory mourning—the parents mourning both for the well child whom they had lost, and for the sick child whose survival was far from certain. All the classic symptoms of grief—sighing, crying, preoccupation with the child, loss of appetite, depression, nervousness and sleep difficulties—were noted. In addition, other symptoms included feelings of tension, headaches, overeating or anorexia, and nervous reactions. Often such symptoms were very pervasive; for example, the mother of a three-year-old said:

'I took bad with my nerves in the summer after she was diagnosed. The doctor I was with wouldn't give me anything. He said just to fight it. I've never been to the stage where I've needed long treatment—but I had one course of tranquillisers for my hands. My jaws were clenched up. I didn't sleep and eat. Now I find I worry a lot more about trivial things quite unrelated to the child—they annoy me more.'

Such symptoms increased if the child was unwell, or needed emergency treatment; thus, one mother commented:

'When he takes ill and goes into hospital the tension would start and build up a bit. I have sleep problems. I can't get to sleep. My mind's working all the time. I keep making tea all the time—especially if I'm here on my own. I feel hungry and I make food.'

Often such symptoms lead to a general irritability and some parents encountered within themselves a bewildering sense of hostility towards the child, the medical personnel who were caring for him, each other, and even their other well children. Such feelings, engendered by the many frustrations implicit in the situation, further confused and depressed them. Thus one mother confided:

> 'Things get on top of me, and I'm off again. I sleep day and night. I shout at him when I'm like this, and ignore him, and then I feel "poor little thing". I shout at my husband as well. It's really just worry over John.'

Often parents attempted to ignore these symptoms, and most endeavoured to avoid troubling their doctors with them. Many expressed views similar to the mother who said: 'I don't run to the doctor too much for myself. I feel I'm imposing when I have to go so much with the child.'

Very occasionally, parents experienced more serious health problems because of worry over the sick child, such as psychiatric disturbance necessitating inpatient treatment, or ulcers. This was the exception rather than the rule, however, and most parents, though subtly and pervasively affected, soldiered on, attempting to do their duty.

4

Understanding the illness

'No one else knows anything about it round here except the
doctor. People don't know of it. We never heard tell of it 'til it
came to our house.'

(Father)

Once told the nature of their child's illness, parents are faced with
the problem of assimilating what for the majority seem complex and
frightening facts. In some instances, where the illness is well
recognised, their difficulties may be accentuated by the gratuitous
comments of family and friends. Often 'information' received from
such sources is sensational, contradictory or erroneous. Thus, for
example, parents of children with cancer may be subjected to horrific
stories regarding treatment procedures and outcome which bear
little relationship to the actual medical facts.

By contrast, parents of children with more obscure disorders,
either those which are numerically rare, or those which have only
recently been identified and labelled, may be handicapped in terms
of their comprehension because of a general lack of knowledge
existent in the community. Rather than having to fend off unwanted
and painfully misleading 'facts', as the previous group of parents
may have to do, these latter parents may find themselves repeatedly
required to explain their child's ailment. Replication often produces
discomfort on their part, and leads to a growing sense of isolation.
They feel they are fighting a lone battle in a non-comprehending
world.

In both instances parent groups can do much to alleviate suffering. By putting parents in touch with each other, by providing well written, simple explanations of the child's illness, and by funding research into the condition, they diminish 'that isolation which accentuates all suffering' (Saunders, 1969). Understandably, many such organisations have sprung up over the past twenty years and most of the well-recognised children's diseases now have active, supportive, parent groups.[1]

Similarly, with cf a group of interested parents and clinicians met together in London in 1964 and founded the Cystic Fibrosis Research Trust, a voluntary organisation which has as its aims: (1) the financing of research to find a complete cure for the disease, and, in the meantime, to improve upon current methods of treatment; (2) the forming of branches and groups throughout the United Kingdom for the purpose of helping and advising parents with the everyday problems of caring for cf children; (3) the education of the public about the disease, and thereby, through increased knowledge, helping to promote earlier diagnosis in young children.

In addition to financing basic research in hospitals and universities throughout the United Kingdom, the Trust produces booklets dealing with every aspect of the disease. It also issues a regular newsletter which keeps parents abreast of latest research developments, new treatment techniques, and fund-raising activities. These publications seem especially useful to parents and the contribution they make to the parents' understanding of the illness will be discussed later in this chapter. Initially, however, parents receive basic information regarding their child's condition from the diagnosing physician, and although this topic was dealt with in chapter 3, a brief recapitulation would seem essential.

Initial reception of information

Whilst most parents felt that the diagnostic interview had been tactfully and kindly handled, it was obvious from their responses that, despite this opportunity to learn, many gaps remained in their knowledge. Mothers generally seemed to have learnt more than fathers, a difference possibly due to (1) their more usual presence, and (2) their possibly greater readiness to receive such information.

[1] A list of some such organisations is included at the end of this book.

Fathers differed in the degree of information they received, differences being related to (1) presence at diagnosis and (2) socio-economic status. Managerial and professional fathers, whether present or not at the diagnostic interview, learnt more than skilled fathers, who in turn learnt more than unskilled fathers, a relationship possibly due to subtle differences in parental role expectation which made the better-educated fathers more ready to receive such information. In addition, the overwhelming sense of shock and emotional turmoil some parents experienced at diagnosis, and their subsequent attempts at warding away threatening facts, contributed to their lack of knowledge.

Often these factors combined to render the parents' post-diagnostic knowledge at best sketchy, at worst non-existent, and it therefore seemed crucial to learn whether this lack was ever redressed. Several possibilities existed. The less well-informed parents, realising their inadequacies, might press for subsequent interviews with medical advisers or search for information on their own. Alternatively, those who were ill-informed at the outset might fail to appreciate the need for further instruction and continue in a state of ignorance. Equally, if lack of knowledge was due solely to denial, and denial persisted, little might be learnt.

Subsequent counselling by medical advisers

In order to evaluate the ways in which parents informed themselves of the disease after the diagnostic interview, questions were put to them concerning their subsequent counselling by medical advisers. Because of the gravity of the illness it was expected that most would have been fully informed concerning causes, symptoms and treatment at some time by either their family doctor or the paediatrician and if this had not occurred at diagnosis, it would occur soon after. Surprisingly, a very substantial proportion of parents—46 per cent of mothers and 74 per cent of fathers—denied that any doctor had ever taken a lot of trouble to explain their child's illness or treatment to them.

The apparent discrepancy between sexes in this respect may in part be attributable to the fact that generally in Ulster it was the mother who accompanied the child for his physical examination or clinic visits, and, as with the diagnostic interview, she was therefore more easily available for subsequent counselling.

In such circumstances an extra effort was required of the father if he was also to be directly informed. As might be predicted on the basis of previous observations regarding the relationship of social class to father's presence at diagnosis (above, p. 36), upon investigation it was found that only the more able or determined fathers eventually obtained a full explanation of the disease. Table 9 shows that whilst 45 per cent of fathers drawn from socio-economic classes I and II felt they were fully informed, only a quarter of class III fathers, and no class IV and V fathers, experienced similar satisfaction.

This apparent relationship between social class and subsequent excellence of counselling by medical advisers may arise in several ways. The more able fathers may comprehend better what is said. Their own greater natural authority may equip them better to question and sift the information given, and therefore obtain a clearer picture of the illness. Similarly, the doctor may be better able to converse with them as social equals, and therefore more able to adjust the flow of information to meet their needs. Perhaps, even more essentially, the more able and determined fathers may be more highly motivated in their quest for knowledge and more willing to present themselves for interview. Thus, in contrast to the semi- and unskilled fathers who seemed keen to dodge the issue or leave it entirely to their wives, managerial and professional fathers clearly viewed understanding the illness as one of their many parental responsibilities.

This supposition was corroborated when parents were asked whether at the time of the survey they would like further and fuller explanations of basic information. Whilst 56 per cent of mothers of all social classes said they would be willing to learn more, Table 9 shows that by contrast to the majority of class I and II fathers, only a third of class III fathers and 12 per cent of class IV and V fathers indicated that they would be willing to learn anything more. This obvious reluctance to understand the illness on the part of the less well educated fathers may be attributable first to their greater unwillingness to assume responsibility, and second, to their more pronounced tendency to deny the implications of the disease. Comments such as the following came up often in the course of the interviews: 'What you don't know you can't worry about'; 'Too much knowledge is not a good thing'; 'Knowing won't help you to care for her'; 'I leave it all to the mammy'.

Table 9 *The father's search for illness information, according to socio-economic class*

	I and II	IIIM and IIINM	IV and V
Illness fully explained to father by medical personnel (%)	45	25	0
Father would welcome further explanations of basic illness facts (%)	63	33	12
Father tried to learn more himself about illness following diagnosis (%)	72	54	50
No.	11	24	8

Perhaps less educated fathers had early learnt to limit their questioning and develop an accepting attitude in order to survive in a society which placed a low premium on their opinions. Alternatively, denial may have flourished where active participation in care and treatment was precluded by convention, and where the father was permitted to avoid the implications of the child's daily existence. In such circumstances, denial may have resulted from a genuine lack of appreciation, or may have emerged reactively to counter feelings of guilt and helplessness occasioned by lack of active care.

Parental search for information

At the outset it seemed reasonable to suppose that most parents would be anxious to understand their child's illness and treatment as well as possible, and where they felt they had not been fully informed by medical advisers, they would themselves seek information. Generally this assumption seemed true. Seventy-four per cent of mothers and 60 per cent of fathers did try and find out more for themselves about the disease. Mothers of all classes were equally enthusiastic in this quest, but, as might be predicted, the more able class I and II fathers were still slightly more zealous than other fathers in this respect (Table 9).

Interestingly, when I looked at the entire group of parents I found that there was a pronounced tendency for those who felt themselves to be fully informed by a medical adviser, to pursue equally enthusiastically additional information on their own.

Thus, Table 10 shows that of the 38 parents who felt the illness had been explained fully to them by a doctor, the majority—31—continued to search subsequently on their own for further information. By contrast, almost half—26—of the 59 parents who felt they

Table 10 *The relationship of extent of medical instruction to parental search for information*

	Parent tried to find out more about illness	*Parent did not search for further information*
Fully informed by medical adviser	31	7
Not fully informed by medical adviser	33	26

were not fully informed by the physician, did nothing further to combat their lack of knowledge.[1] These relationships may occur for different reasons, for example, parents who are fully informed initially by a concerned physician may later respond to his concern by seeking information on their own. In this respect their already full discussions may arm them both emotionally and intellectually for their task of finding out. They may feel more confident subsequently in this task, no longer being afraid of the unknown. Equally, it could be that those who are highly motivated to gain knowledge, seize upon or make suitable opportunities to do so, whether these be with the doctor, other parents, friends, or medical literature. By contrast, those who are afraid to find out defend themselves from knowledge whenever and however it presents itself.

Sources of information

As mentioned previously some parents find difficulty in accurately informing themselves about their child's illness. Popular comment

---

[1] Differences between groups were assessed using the χ^2 test.
$\chi^2 = 5.6788$, df $= 1$, $p < 0.02$.

can be erroneous or painfully misleading, or alternatively, non-existent, where the disease is relatively uncommon. As a consequence many parents turn anxiously to medical dictionaries or write to health magazines. One of the most useful sources of information—and one especially devised for parents—is the range of pamphlets concerning the disease and its treatment, published by an appropriate charitable organisation. In terms of cf, this literature is written for parents and supplied on request by the CF Research Trust.[1]

In order to assess the usefulness of this source of information, parents were asked whether they had ever seen any of these booklets, how they were recommended to them, and how useful they had found them to be.

Eighty per cent of mothers and 68 per cent of fathers said they had read some of these pamphlets. Interestingly, in some families only one parent studied this literature, the other parent declining to do so—this avoidance reaction often being due to a deep-seated need to deny the reality of the disease. Generally, as with other sources of information, mothers showed a greater willingness to inform themselves in this way.

Frequently, parents had been put in touch with the Trust by the diagnosing physician. Sometimes referral had been made through an interested health visitor or district nurse. Occasionally the parent was first contacted by a member of the local CF Parents' Association Committee, who, upon gaining permission, forwarded his name to the Trust.

Eighty-three per cent of all parents who had read the relevant literature found it helpful. Generally it was praised for the simplicity of the language used, the clarity of the illustrations, the variety of informative facts provided, and most especially for the aura of optimism which it emanated. Parents frequently commented that the pamphlets were the only optimistic source of information which they had encountered and as such gave them hope and encouragement to continue in their task of treating the child.

One father said: 'We find them very instructive and very encouraging.' Another man added: 'One thing that is reassuring is seeing teenagers doing things that one would expect of normal teenagers and that is reassuring, and knowing that there is a Trust, and it is financing research on a large scale.'

[1] The national headquarters of this organisation are at 5 Blyth Road, Bromley, Kent.

This latter point was stressed by many who found it hopeful to be reminded of continuing research efforts and improving treatment techniques, which might benefit not only their own child but other similarly affected children.

Perhaps the highest accolade of praise came from a father who said that by contrast to mass media reports of the illness, which they hoped people would ignore, they regularly passed on CF Trust pamphlets to their wider family and friends.

Those few parents who had read the CF Trust literature and found it distressing usually did so because, by being honest, the pamphlets eroded their attempts at denial. Comments such as the following were made:

'At the time I was first told I was given pamphlets, but my GP tore them up. They were alarming and they said she might never be able to go to a normal school, and they were dubious whether inoculations should be started'.

Another mother added: 'They confused me a bit. They said a few things like "not living", which were different from my doctor.'

Eighty per cent of mothers and 66 per cent of fathers said they wished they had been given the CF Trust pamphlets to read at the time they were first told of their child's illness. They offered many reasons to explain the value of such a service to them. For many, having something to read would have surmounted the difficulties experienced initially, due to shock, in comprehending what was said. For example, one mother reported: 'You can take things in better if you sit and read it on your own. If someone is telling you a lot it goes over your head.'

Other points stressed were (1) reading material could be referred to by fathers in leisure time, thereby obviating 'waste' of valuable working time; (2) the pamphlets provided a basis for subsequent questioning of the doctor, giving the parents a sense of personal authority, and introducing them to medical terms which were often used during clinical interviews and which they had previously found difficult to understand or recall; (3) it provided facts for those parents who were either too reticent or uncertain to question their doctor, or for parents whose doctor was too evasive to be questioned. As one mother expressed it: 'You just were told, and that was that. Just told and you had no way of finding out, and if the GP wouldn't talk you had no one to ask of it.'

A father who felt CF Trust pamphlets would have been especially valuable following diagnosis said: 'I couldn't get myself to ask him. I wasn't the type that could probe or question.'

Alternatively, those parents who were glad not to have received literature to read following the diagnosis either said they had been told enough initially, for example, 'I thought he explained it in such detail. Whatever he told us was just conveyed into the mind and it stayed there;' or, they were continually trying to deny the severity of the disease in an attempt to cope with the overwhelming threat it posed. Thus one father commented: 'I was very nervous then. I wouldn't have coped if I'd had the true facts. I would have taken it worse.' A mother added: 'I prefer to know as little as possible about it. This may be the wrong attitude but it is how I feel. Possibly if I knew I'd be too discouraged.'

Occasionally parents argued for a time lag between being told the diagnosis and being given all the relevant facts. They felt that an over-frank presentation at the outset would have been disastrous for them, but accepted that in the long term, honesty was desirable. 'I think reading it then would have been too soon. You try to forget it. You don't want to study too much.' 'I couldn't have accepted it then, but I've learnt to live with it now, and I could read it now, but not then.'

Information gleaned from the mass media

A further possible source of information was that provided by the mass media—either articles in the press or television programmes. Seventy-five per cent of mothers and 55 per cent of fathers had either read an article about the disease in the newspapers or seen a television programme devoted to it. In contrast to the generally positive response to CF Research Trust literature, exactly half the parents who had been subjected to accounts of cf by the mass media found them lacking or erroneous. 'Hurtful and untrue', 'exaggerating', 'very frightening' and 'misinformed' were terms used to describe such presentations. Some parents felt that their handicaps were being exploited in order to give the media a good story, or to help some would-be fund raiser to accomplish his aims. To quote their comments: 'It was a lot of codswallop to put it plainly. For the press it's a story at all costs.' 'They painted too gloomy a picture.

Something to do with raising money, and the only way you can do that is to get sympathy.'

One mother read an article in a paper captioned 'These children will die'. She said: 'It was very heartless. I just sat and wept. It was not very tactful at all. I know they have to get sympathy but from the parents' point of view it's not nice to open a paper and read that sort of thing.'

Frequently reports raised hopes, only to dash them later. For example, several suggested that a cure had been found, and one claimed that a test had been devised to detect the disease during pregnancy. Parents bitterly resented being misled in this way. Similarly, they resented the overwhelmingly pessimistic tone of some articles and programmes, not only because these challenged their own optimism, but also because sick children might be inadvertently subjected to them.

One mother, whose ten-year-old son had seen such a programme on television commented:

'He saw this programme on television. It said some children were going to die. He said, "That doesn't mean me, does it, Mum?" Then I had to tell him that some children who have it are very, very bad, and some children do die. I explained that it was the chest that was the problem and his was clear and he accepted it. Never mentioned it again—just carried on playing.'

Rating the usefulness of sources of information

Parents were asked to assess the helpfulness of the different sources of knowledge they had encountered (Table 11).

For mothers the paediatrician was most often thought to be of help in understanding the disease, whilst fathers clearly found written material to be of more value. Such differences are explicable in terms of the degree of contact between the individuals concerned, mothers being more available for verbal instruction from medical advisers, fathers relying more heavily on leisure reading.

Generally, other sources of possible information were dismissed as being unhelpful where they were unduly pessimistic, for example one mother who had lost two previous children found her own family, her health visitor and her GP of no value whatsoever because: 'They just say there's no future for him. They say "it's

Table 11 *Sources of information deemed of 'very much' or 'moderate' help in understanding cf*

	Mothers (%)	Fathers (%)
Paediatrician	69	39
Books (including cf pamphlets)	60	51
CF Trust (lectures, parents' meetings, personnel)	34	33
GP	22	13
Family	12	8
Friends	2	6
No.	52	45

going to come some day sooner or later and you must just get that into your mind".' After such conversations this mother felt suicidal: 'They just say God should have taken him at nine weeks and I shouldn't go on nursing him.' Even the clergy were of little help in her distress: 'They're very sympathetic but they don't understand. They just say "if God does take him, we'll know where he is".'

On the other hand, some parents found themselves cut off from sources of information or comfort by the denial processes of others. Relatives and friends were made too uncomfortable by the threatening aspects of the disease to be able to discuss the child's progress or treatment realistically. They therefore tended to deny reality—forming what Friedman *et al.* (1963) has termed 'concentric circles of disbelief'. Thus they were of little help to parents in understanding the disease. For example, one mother commented of her family: 'They just say, "maybe she'll grow out of it," and I know she won't.'

What was clearly essential in family contacts was a balance of honesty and optimism. Often parents were tired of explaining the disease over and over again. Because of the general ignorance concerning it in the community, they found themselves more often in the role of teacher rather than taught, and this was both isolating and wearisome. As one father commented: 'No one else knows anything about it round here except the doctor. People don't know of it. We never heard tell of it 'til it came to our house.'

Occasionally parents of other sick children could be of value, though some parents found such contact a mixed blessing, highlighting their own shortcomings. As one mother said: 'They're not really a help. They're more of a hindrance. They worried me more. They gave me a guilt complex.'

Often parents met each other in an informal, unstructured fashion which, though conducive to the development of friendships, could also maximise the sharing of anxieties. In addition, the development and expression of compensatory one-up-man-ship in the more insecure parents could undermine the wellbeing of others. Perhaps such parent contacts are most helpful when formally convened and positively channelled, as in the case of CF Trust parents' meetings, where all come together for the sharing of information and opinion, but where the discussion is optimistically orientated.

Parental understanding of the illness

Finally, before leaving the subject, it seemed necessary to evaluate, albeit crudely, the actual extent of the parents' knowledge concerning the disease. Rather than question parents on all aspects of the illness, it was decided to concentrate on assessing their comprehension of one of the most complex aspects—the genetic nature of the illness. Parents were therefore asked to explain what they understood of the chances of their children's children having the disease.

The responses made were graded into categories, according to the completeness of the parents' understanding. Excellent or good responses were those in which there was some appreciation of the nature of recessive inheritance, with the implications of 'equal responsibility' of both parents, and where the parents were able to evaluate realistically the chances of their affected child reproducing normally. Moderate to poor understanding included responses indicative of some, but generally a less complete, understanding of the genetic risks involved, and the nil category included responses which indicated that parents knew nothing about this contingency.

Twenty per cent of parents had an excellent/good understanding, 60 per cent had a moderate/poor understanding, and 20 per cent claimed to know nothing of this aspect of their child's disease.

When an analysis of these results was made according to sex and social class certain trends were apparent (Table 12).

Generally, as might be expected on the basis of the preceding discussion, mothers had a better understanding of the genetic aspects of the illness than fathers, though as a group, social class I

Table 12 *Degree of understanding of illness, according to sex and social class of parent*

		I and II (%)	III M and III NM (%)	IV and V (%)
Mothers	Excellent/good understanding	28	11	18
	Moderate understanding	58	63	73
	Nil	14	26	9
	No.	14	26	11
Fathers	Excellent/good understanding	45	12	12
	Moderate understanding	37	55	52
	Nil	18	33	36
	No.	11	24	8

and II fathers had the best overall comprehension. By contrast, over a third of the skilled, semi-skilled and unskilled fathers had no real knowledge of the illness.

These findings were confirmed in another way. When school leaving age of parents was correlated with degree of understanding a significant difference emerged between the school leaving age of parents in each of the three understanding groups (Table 13). The longer the parents remained in school the better their understanding of the genetic risks attendant on cf.[1]

Interestingly, those parents who said that a doctor had taken a lot of trouble to explain the illness fully to them, tended to have a better understanding of the genetics than parents who were not fully informed by their doctor.[2] This relationship may in part be due to the zeal of the doctor in imparting such information, and also the the fact

---

[1] Differences in the mothers' school leaving age between the excellent/good and the nil groups, and between the excellent/good and the moderate groups attained significance at the 0·05 level, using the t test. Similarly, differences in the fathers' school leaving age between the excellent/good and the nil group, and the moderate /poor and the nil groups were significant at the 0·05 level, using the t test.

[2] Differences between groups were assessed using χ^2 test. $\chi^2 = 8·18$, df $= 3$, $p < 0·05$.

Table 13 *Average school-leaving age of parents in each of the three understanding groups*

		Excellent/good	Moderate/poor	Nil
Mothers	Age	16·1	14·10	14·3
	No.	10	33	9
Fathers	Age	15·3	15·2	14·0
	No.	9	23	13

that parents who are fully informed in this way usually make it their business to search out additional sources of information. This supposition was confirmed by the fact that the twenty-six fathers who did try and find out more about the illness on their own had a significantly better comprehension of the genetic risks than the seventeen fathers who made no effort.[1]

Summary

It seems safe to conclude that there are considerable individual differences in the enthusiasm with which parents pursue knowledge concerning their child's condition. Generally, in Northern Ireland mothers were more keen to acquire information than fathers, and this may be due partly to their role expectation, and partly to the greater need they have for such information. In this community it is usually the mother whose responsibility it is to look after and administer treatment to the sick child (see below, p. 82). In addition, managerial and professional fathers show an equally well developed enthusiasm for gaining knowledge about their child's condition, being more often present at diagnosis, receiving more counselling subsequently by medical personnel and being more willing to receive further explanations concerning basic facts than fathers from other occupational levels. These differences may also be attributable to role expectation, fathers in the higher social classes tending to support their wives more in these tasks, and aspiring to greater mutuality as parents.

Generally, those who are willing to learn seem able to do so, be it either by direct confrontation with medical personnel or indirectly

[1] Differences between groups were assessed using the t test. t = 2·88, df = 41, p < 0·01.

through perusing relevant literature or joining a parent group. Conversely, those who do not seize one type of opportunity to inform themselves generally seem unwilling to take another, and often their tardiness in this respect seems more directly attributable to their own wish to deny the illness, rather than to any lack of suitable encouragement on the part of caring personnel. The most frequent tendencies to denial were found in the ranks of the skilled, semi-skilled, and unskilled fathers, perhaps due to the fact that these fathers can most easily persist in denial, rarely being called upon to involve themselves actively in the sick child's care or treatment.

5

Coping with an inherited disease

'I suppose we are responsible in a sense—genetically responsible —but the problem here is, had we known we were carriers we would have made the decision not to have children—but we didn't know we were carriers.'

(Father)

When parents of sick children come to appreciate that the illness is inherited, their personal distress is maximised. Feelings of guilt are accentuated, for parents both see themselves as failures in terms of preventing the disease and also feel themselves responsible for it. Their already diminished self-esteem may be lowered yet further by the intrusive comments of close relatives, who themselves feel implicated and become anxious to assess the exact genetic facts. Perhaps most hurtful of all, at a time when one of their children is threatened and they are being forced to re-evaluate their hopes and expectations for this child, parents must also consider the desirability of limiting further conception.

Several issues must be evaluated before any proper decision can be reached. First, parents must discover the risk of repetition. Second, they must assess the degree of burden imposed by the illness both upon the child and upon the family unit as a whole, and, finally, they must discover whether a reliable intra-uterine test is available to predict recurrence in subsequent pregnancy.

Inherited diseases differ widely in all these respects. With some, the risk of repetition may be exceedingly slight; with others, it may be as high as one in two. Similarly, the degree of burden varies enormously. Some children may be utterly incapacitated, mentally or physically, by their disorder, whilst others may lead a relatively normal life. Equally, in some conditions such as mongolism, it is now possible to predict recurrence accurately during the first few weeks of any subsequent pregnancy, in which event, if desired, termination can occur. In other conditions there is still no accurate pre-natal screening test.

As yet, no one fully knows how these factors influence the parents' decision with regard to family planning, though it would seem logical to assume that the couple faced with a minimal risk, low burden, easily predicted condition, might more willingly chance further pregnancy in the hope of completing their family than parents faced with a high risk, high burden, non-predictable disease. It may also be relevant to consider the nature of the resultant disorder, whether mental or physical.

Similarly, decision-making may be influenced by personal factors such as the size of the existing family, the presence or absence of well children, and the degree of parental understanding of the genetic risks. Family limitation may be less of a problem in families in which the sick child comes low in birth order and previous children are well. By contrast, couples whose first child is sick, and who have no other children, may experience greater discomfort in limiting their family. Similarly, parents with religious or personal scruples concerning birth control would seem especially disadvantaged.

In order to evaluate some of the factors which influence family planning decisions, questions were included relating to this topic when talking to study parents.

Although, generally, people know little about cf, it is in fact the most common genetic disorder in north-west Europe with approximately one in twenty of us carrying the abnormal gene which produces the disorder. Few of us are aware of this for carriers do not have the disease, and unfortunately at the present time there is no means of detecting the presence of the abnormal gene in the apparently healthy carrier. Cf is a recessive disorder, which means that to produce the disease two abnormal genes are necessary—one inherited from each parent. Consequently, all marriages between carriers are at risk in terms of the disease. On average, in our community, such marriages occur at the rate of one in every 400. All children of such marriages have a one in four chance of inheriting the disease. Generally, where there are several children in an affected family, some have the disease, some carry the faulty gene and, though healthy themselves, are capable of transmitting the disorder to future generations, and others are well children, neither carriers nor having the disease. Figure 1 shows the classical pattern of recessive inheritance (the lined oblong representing the faulty

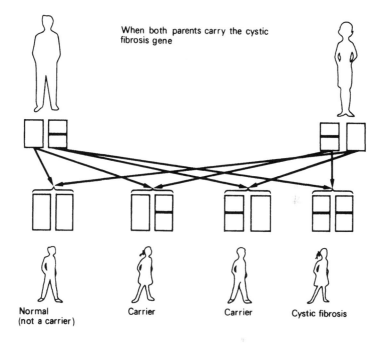

When both parents carry the cystic fibrosis gene

Normal (not a carrier) Carrier Carrier Cystic fibrosis

Figure 1   *The classic pattern of cf inheritance*

gene). In this imaginary family, one out of the four children is affected, two are carriers, and one is healthy. However, this is only a statistical model, based on an immense sample, and does not apply to every family unit. Thus, in some families there are no well children and all the children have the disease. Similarly, in some families all the apparently healthy children may be carriers—though, as no test is yet available to detect carriers, it is not possible to state this with certainty.

Before any family planning decisions can be reached, it is obviously essential for parents to appreciate the genetic risks. Parents are often handicapped in this task by the complexity of the genetic terminology and the unfamiliarity of the concepts used.

Words such as genes, genetic, recessive, inheritance and carriers were seldom fully understood—a factor also noted by McCrae *et al.* (1973) in Scotland and Leonard *et al.* (1972) in the USA, and this produced considerable resultant confusion in the parents' comprehension. For example, a semi-skilled father said: 'It isn't really an inherited condition but it does come from the parents—both parents having the same genetic fault.' The wife of a labourer believed: 'I have a genie inside me that sometimes causes the disease.'

Parents found it difficult to understand the recessive nature of the disease and the fact that, on average, only one in four of their children would be affected. Their comments express their general bewilderment. Thus a mother confided:

'It comes through one side of the family or the other. Not through both sides. They said it would be in the first child, then skip one—coming again—then skip one. How doesn't it come in the two?'

Estimates regarding risk of recurrence in subsequent pregnancies were often wildly inaccurate, ranging from 50:50 to one in a million. Similarly, estimates regarding the genetic risks to future generations were rarely understood. Thus a skilled father said: 'The chances are a thousand to one that my children will meet up with someone with the same fault in their system.'

Often the parents' own vague physiological notions were incorporated into their overall understanding, producing additional complications, for example: 'The doctor explained to me that it had something to do with the blood group and the two persons' bodies.'

Confusion concerning genetic terminology was also seen in a recent North American study (Leonard *et al.*, 1972) which discovered that 44 per cent of sixty-one families given personal genetic counselling by the authors had imperfectly understood the information they were given.

Despite such difficulties, however, most parents had achieved a moderate understanding of the genetic risks involved in the disease by the time of this study. This understanding was attained despite the fact that 70 per cent of fathers and 25 per cent of mothers claimed not to have been given genetic information at diagnosis, and 46 per cent of mothers and 74 per cent of fathers denied having the illness explained fully to them by any doctor.

Understanding of the genetic risks was best, as one might expect, amongst the class I and II fathers, though mothers from other socio-economic classes had a better understanding than their husbands (see above, p. 62). Parents of both sexes who stayed at school beyond the statutory school-leaving age knew more about genetics than other less educated parents. Similarly, those parents knew most whose doctor had taken a lot of trouble to explain the illness fully to them, or who had taken trouble to inform themselves.

In the context of illness understanding, it seemed possible to identify two very different parent groups. On the one hand, there were those who were often most able educationally and professionally, and who pursued knowledge relentlessly. On the other hand, there were those, often disadvantaged educationally and in terms of their work, who shrank from knowledge however it presented itself, and who were therefore least well informed. Whilst, generally, the two groups were mutually exclusive there existed the occasional class I or II father who preferred to deny reality and could not accept information. Similarly, the exceptional semi-skilled father showed great determination in informing himself and in assisting his wife in the care of the child. Such differences are probably due to previous life circumstances or psycho-dynamic factors as yet not properly understood.

Usually those who were best informed considered family planning more carefully than those with little knowledge. Thus, it was generally the most able parents who did so.

Family-planning advice for parents

Table 14 shows that, while three-quarters of class I, II and III mothers had discussed family planning with a doctor, only a third of class IV and V mothers had done so. Similarly, almost three times as many class I, II and III fathers had done so compared with class IV and V fathers.

Table 14 *Parents who discussed family planning with a doctor,
according to sex and social class*

		I and II	III M and III NM	IV and V
Mothers	%	78	75	36
	No.	14	26	11
Fathers	%	36	43	12
	No.	11	24	8

One might suppose that families who already had a history of cf
prior to the birth of the child under study would seek, or have
received, more family planning advice than families who were
meeting the illness for the first time, but this was not so. Upon
investigation it was found that mothers and fathers who were
coping with the illness for the first time received proportionately
more help in terms of family planning advice than parents who
already had another living cf child, or who had previously lost one
with the disease.

Occasionally, this surprisingly low level of family planning discussion in families with previous history of disease could be attributed
to the fact that the physicians involved, by virtue of the existing
family history, presumed such counselling had taken place at the
time of the first diagnosis. Any later repetition therefore seemed
gratuitous. Thus a class I mother, who had lost a previous baby with
cf, commented:

> 'They explained the genetics with the first baby. But that time
> was a wee bit of a blur. Bits of it are a haze. Definitely, that
> was a part of my life which is blotted out, and I would presume
> that the doctor did talk at that stage, and then presumed that
> she wouldn't have to talk again about it after this new baby.'

A further possibility is that parents with a previous history of the
disease felt more distress concerning it, and therefore developed an
exaggerated tendency to defend themselves from reality through
denial. Thus they avoided situations in which their sense of responsibility was accentuated. About 16 per cent of parents who had
never discussed family planning with a doctor had never talked it
over with anyone else—not even their spouse. Assessing such
families carefully, one is forced to conclude that some previous

history of infant loss may accentuate this reticence, so also may low intelligence or an already strained marital relationship. Often these factors were interrelated.

To take an example. Mr G. was a highly intelligent professional man with a family of four children. His first child had died of cf whilst an infant. At this time Mrs G. became greatly disturbed and engaged in suicidal acts such as flinging the car door open whilst the vehicle was moving, and trying to jump out. Whether to combat his wife's distress, or because of his own despair, Mr G. refused to talk of the infant's death and pretended nothing had happened. Although both parents were probably given genetic counselling at this time, and Mr G. had easy access to genetic information, they continued to have children. At no time would Mr G. discuss the necessity for family limitation, even after a second cf child was born. Sixteen years after the original loss, and ten years after the birth of the next affected child, he was still refusing to talk, even about transitory symptoms or daily treatment. Mrs G. was deeply distressed by this and divided in her loyalties. She did not know whether to counsel the child regarding the illness, which would annoy her husband, or to ignore the matter, as he did. Her resultant tension was considerable, and she regarded her marriage as most unsatisfactory. Possibly as a reaction to family silence and tension, the affected child was exhibiting a syndrome of protest and denial behaviour, refusing necessary treatments, all hospital and dental visits, and crying for reassurance about peripheral activities. Despite this the Gs continued to have further children.

Stresses occasioned for parents by the genetic nature of the disease

A sense of guilt and responsibility   Apart from the many stresses associated with the chronic, and potentially fatal, nature of the disease, parents were asked whether the inherited nature of the illness had produced any special stress for them; in particular, whether it had exaggerated any feelings of guilt and responsibility they might have.

While the majority of parents denied such feelings, seeing the illness as a chance happening, something which could neither have been predicted nor avoided, 36 per cent of mothers and 24 per cent of fathers admitted that they did feel guilty because they were transmitters of disease to their children. Thus a skilled father explained:

'My first reaction on being told was to remember that my mother had told me two cousins had died of it, and I blamed myself for not thinking of it. For otherwise I would never have got married. I only thought then that it was from my side of the family. I didn't realise it needed two. I felt very bitter about it. I worried a lot. I went up to my family that night and felt very bad about it. I haven't got over that feeling yet.'

Whilst, generally, mothers felt more sense of guilt and responsibility than fathers, two further factors appeared to affect the extent of these feelings. The first was social class. The second was previous experience with the illness.

Table 15 shows that, with the exception of class IV and V mothers, there was a tendency for the higher socio-economic groupings to experience proportionately more feelings of guilt and

Table 15 *Parents experiencing feelings of guilt and responsibility, according to sex and social class*

		I and II	III M and III NM	IV and V
Mothers	%	46	21	63
	No.	14	26	11
Fathers	%	33	21	12
	No.	11	24	8
Total		25	50	19

responsibility. Similarly, 50 per cent of the mothers who had some knowledge of the illness prior to the birth of the study child experienced feelings of guilt and responsibility as compared with only 26 per cent of mothers who had no previous knowledge of the illness. Presumably the more able and knowledgeable parents felt, rightly or wrongly, that they should have known and prevented the illness occurring. Thus one young professional father commented:

'I do feel a bit responsible. I suppose if there had been twenty years' further research I would have known. Everyone would have been screened before they married, and we would have been warned of the chances.'

A mother of three cf children, who had never practised birth control and denied being given family planning advice, said:

'I've often thought—well, if they hadn't been born, if the doctor had said, "You shouldn't have any more for your sake or the children's," then it wouldn't have been a sin. There wouldn't have been any more. It just keeps coming back and forward in my mind. It keeps coming back and it fades away again. I just kept getting pregnant before I could do anything about it.'

A young mother, who had lost a previous child, said: 'I was responsible. If I'd known with the first one that there was a chance with the next, I wouldn't have had any more children.'

Such comments speak very eloquently for the enormous need to fully advise parents at diagnosis regarding risk of recurrence.

Occasionally, parents appeared to have dwelt on their guilt considerably over time and had evolved elaborate theories implicating their own inadequacies to explain the occurrence of the disease in their children. For example, a deeply religious professional man confided:

'Sometimes I've wondered whether her condition had some personal relationship with my relationship with God—sort of a chastening thing—not punishment—just a chastening experience. I still feel this. It doesn't worry me, for the thing is fixed now. I would never look for healing on her part—what they call divine healing—for I feel it has to be that way—it's the result of my failing, sort of.'

The mother of a big family whose child was reared largely in hospital saw the disease occurring as a result of her supposed negligence:

'Well, I didn't actually cause the disease for I've never done anything in my life, but somehow his not being reared with me, his being reared in hospital not like the other children, I felt I didn't care as much for the one that was out of the house. Maybe I'm doing wrong and getting paid for these things.'

Feelings of personal inadequacy and worthlessness Feelings of guilt accentuated feelings of personal inadequacy and worthlessness, making the parents question their own value as people and parents.

Thus a young skilled father commented: 'I'm right and healthy and was a PT instructor in the army, and that's what made me think, how could I produce a child with such a disease?' The mother of a first baby said: 'I did feel guilty at the start. I remember I did feel sometimes it must have been my fault she was like that. I just imagined all babies were healthy and if they're not it must be your fault.'

Such thoughts could be exaggerated by the unthinkingly cruel and intrusive questions and comments of neighbours and relatives—especially grandparents, many of whom were anxious to establish a 'blame' for the illness on the other side of the house. As one mother put it: 'We came home and told my father. He said, "It must come from him—only from him. There's nothing wrong with you."'
Another mother said: 'My parents saw it as a personal insult—their having something and passing it on.' Often parents were made extremely unhappy by such unthinking attempts at denial.

Anger and resentment towards the spouse Occasionally, where there was an inadequate understanding of recessive inheritance, parents felt angry and resentful towards their marital partner, in the mistaken belief that the disease was entirely inherited from them. Fortunately, only a few parents—10 per cent of women and 5 per cent of men—persisted in such beliefs, although a greater number reported that they had initially felt this way. Often such feelings were very corrosive, negatively influencing the marriage. Thus a mother who had lost two previous infants, and frequently felt suicidal, said:

'I can't let it outright to him—but indeed I have felt that way. I know there's a headstone up to his mother and father and it says "a daughter Amanda who died in infancy", but I don't like to put it plain. His mother and father were first cousins—but he wouldn't tell you these things.'

The wife of a manual worker said:

'When I came home I explained it to my husband and my husband was on edge to know which side of the family it was coming from and he said it couldn't be his side, but I accepted it for my father was bronchial and one of his brothers has TB and one of their children died of bronchial pneumonia at eighteen months, and I thought, how do you know it was bronchial pneumonia—it could have been cf.'

Many parents who had received adequate genetic counselling, and had overcome any latent resentment, spontaneously admitted that they were glad both husband and wife shared equal genetic responsibility for cf. Thus a mother who had lost two previous children said:

'I was glad to hear the two of us were carriers of it, because I could never turn on my husband and accuse him. Many times I've joked though—if I had married someone else it would have been all right—because I love children.'

While mothers admitted to experiencing such feelings of resentment and guilt more often than fathers, they seemed better able to expiate it in active caring for the child. Erosive guilt feelings were also lessened by developing a sense of perspective with regard to the child's illness. Parents comforted themselves by thinking of the alternatives. For example: 'If he was blind or dumb, he'd be a lot worse, and he's a very sensible child, and it's something to be thankful for.'

Knowledge of disease prior to the birth of the sick child

A further source of stress for parents was the knowledge of the inherited nature of the disease prior to the birth of the sick child. As outlined in chapter 2, in 41 per cent of cases the parents knew something of the disease prior to the birth of this affected child, and in half of these cases the mother became continuously afraid throughout pregnancy, being convinced that the baby she was carrying would have the disease. In several instances the mother requested an abortion at this stage, but was refused either on medical grounds or because she was thought to be 'fussing unnecessarily'.

Fear of pregnancy

Once told the genetic nature of the disease, many mothers became markedly afraid of having another child. In all, 65 per cent of mothers of child-bearing age reported such fears. Comments such as the following were typical: 'I'd die if I had to go through it again.' 'I'd spend the nine months worrying.' Fear of pregnancy seemed exaggerated by experience of previous loss and also by full comprehension of the genetic risks involved. Thus, whilst two-thirds of the class I, II and III mothers were afraid, only a quarter of mothers from classes IV and V felt similarly. Again, 68 per cent of mothers with a previous knowledge of cf feared pregnancy, as against 45 per cent of mothers with no previous illness history.

Similarly, when the Northern Irish mothers were compared with a comparable group studied in the east of Scotland, they exhibited significantly more fear of pregnancy (Burton *et al.,* 1972)*[1]. In contrast to the Scottish mothers, the Northern Irish mothers had experienced twice as much infant mortality—18 per cent as against 9 per cent—and they displayed a significantly better comprehension of the genetic risks involved.[2] Interestingly, fears of pregnancy seemed to bear little relationship to the method of contraception used. Most of the mothers who avowed themselves afraid were using adequate contraception.

Understandably, fears of pregnancy contributed significantly to a sense of strain in marriage. Of those study mothers who were afraid of pregnancy, over two-thirds said they were experiencing severe strain in their marriage.[3]

Decisions regarding family limitation

Obviously, for many reasons, most parents—84 per cent of mothers and 76 per cent of fathers—felt that they would prefer to limit their family after being told of the genetic risks involved in the illness. This was especially true for parents who had lost previous children, or who had two living affected children. Many reasons were given to explain such decision-making. Some parents stressed their own anguish: 'I could never go through what I have gone through again.' 'Another sick child would kill me.' Others emphasised the needs of the child: 'This one needs all our care.' 'I would feel very guilty now.

* Differences between groups were assessed using the χ^2 test (df $= 1$ unless actually stated).

[1] $\chi^2 = 24\cdot8$, p $< 0\cdot001$.

[2] $\chi^2 = 31\cdot4$, df $= 2$, p $< 0\cdot001$.

[3] $\chi^2 = 6.40$, p $< 0\cdot02$.

I would dread the nine months' waiting.' 'I wouldn't want other children to have it, it wouldn't be fair to the child.'

Occasionally parents cited other reasons to explain the desirability of future family limitation; chief amongst these was the presence of other well children in the family. Mothers stressed that another sick child would prejudice the general wellbeing of all family members. Generally, the larger the existing family, the easier it seemed for the mother to decide upon family limitation.

Similarly, family limitation seemed most easily decided upon and effected where there were no religious scruples concerning contraception. In this respect the twenty-five Catholic mothers in this study experienced especial difficulty. Whilst no Protestant mothers experienced religious difficulties in using contraception, 44 per cent of Catholic mothers felt that contraception created religious problems for them, and they therefore relied on either the 'safe period' or abstinence. In turn, these practices often created considerable stress in their marriage and greatly increased their fear of pregnancy. In addition, over a quarter of the Catholic mothers who used contraception had experienced difficulty in obtaining advice or being given permission to limit their families. Some had to go to a missionary, rather than their parish priest, for permission. Others had difficulties with their family doctors who were also Catholic. For example, one mother was initially put on the pill by her GP only to have her prescription withheld after the Papal Encyclical on the subject.[1] Another mother went to her GP asking to be fitted with a coil. He refused, saying it was against her religion and she must 'go on a chart'. She did and conceived a second affected baby within months.

Resulting marital strain

Naturally, decisions regarding family limitation, difficulties encountered in obtaining adequate contraceptive advice, and the fear of producing another affected child had repercussions on the marital relationship of the couples involved. Twenty per cent of the women and 10 per cent of the men felt their sexual life had been damaged or destroyed by genetic hazards attendant on the disease. This seemed especially true during the earlier years of the child's life, or before

[1] *Humanae Vitae*, 1968.

adequate contraceptive measures were used. Thus one mother commented: 'At the beginning I found I couldn't relax. It wasn't a matter of fearing pregnancy, but psychologically I felt I couldn't relax—my feelings were kind of strung up.' Another mother commented: 'At the beginning I couldn't make love for four years. I was so taut, and with the fear of pregnancy I couldn't relax.' Of love-making, one mother confided: 'I can't be with it, and then I feel I'm letting him down.'

Strain was experienced also in the wider relationship and half the women and 16 per cent of the men said that their marriage was strained. Generally, mothers who reported such stress in marriage were: (1) those who experienced guilt or responsibility for transmitting disease to the child;*[1] (2) those who reported experiencing an unsatisfactory physical relationship with their husbands;[2] (3) those who had been afraid during their pregnancy—very frequently this fear being due to their existent knowledge of the disease;[3] (4) those who had lost previous children. Of the mothers who reported themselves strained, exactly half had lost one or more previous children.[4]

There was also a tendency for mothers reporting strain to be unable to communicate fully with their husbands, to experience religious conflicts over birth control, and to have experienced anger or resentment over their husband's part in the causation of the disease.

One is left with the impression that, where a disease is inherited, the parents' resultant emotional and physical distress is maximised.

* The significance of these relationships was assessed using the χ^2 test (df = 1).
[1] $\chi^2 = 4.52$, $p < 0.05$.
[2] $\chi^2 = 6.3$, $p < 0.02$.
[3] $\chi^2 = 6.40$, $p < 0.02$.
[4] $\chi^2 = 3.85$, $p < 0.05$.

6

Giving the child his treatment

'Looking after him was the most satisfying thing in my life. He was so frail at first. Then I went overboard with treatment, and he put on a huge amount of weight. Yet I felt that all those harsh treatments must wear him down. I felt so guilty giving him that treatment because at that age I couldn't give him any explanation. I played with him afterwards for half an hour but I felt he would think I was a monster.'

(Mother)

Most parents of sick children find themselves involved in helping with treatment aimed at alleviating their child's symptoms. Occasionally, such treatment is hospital-based with the parent playing only a secondary role in supporting the child whilst medical personnel administer therapy. Increasingly, however, with chronically ill children, home management is preferred, with the parents themselves shouldering the full burden of the child's care. Generally, the need for such care is appreciated by the parents, and most accept the task willingly, viewing it as a challenge and finding in it a means of restoring their own shattered self-confidence.

In this way, active participation in the child's treatment programme mobilises parental hope and diminishes feelings of guilt and shame fostered by the diagnosis. The parents' sense of protecting and nurturing their child is re-emphasised and personal esteem is thereby increased. In addition, by affording parents the opportunity to do something positive for the child, requiring regular activity and planning, treatment controls otherwise overwhelming anxiety and helplessness. Because of this, many clinicians (Friedman *et al.,* 1963; Knudson and Natterson, 1960) have noted the way in which active participation in treatment, even though hospital-based, can help parents to adapt to the illness.

Obviously, as with any other regular commitment, treatment can tax the strength and coping abilities of the parents concerned, a factor noted by Turk in her study of cf families (1964). However, as Henley and Albam (1955) suggest when describing parents of children with muscular dystrophy, the personal satisfactions afforded by such care may more than compensate for the strain imposed.

More subtle difficulties may arise, however. For example, by accepting full responsibility for the child's daily care, parents may feel implicated in the illness outcome, and if the child fails to thrive despite their endeavours they may feel doubly guilty. Some parents, despite full intellectual understanding of the necessity for constant care, and apparent acceptance of the task may find difficulties in complying with the required regime. Their consequent sense of guilt may produce tensions in relationships with other caring personnel. Similarly, some parents may become disturbed because they feel they are adding to their child's distress, and they may thus be tempted to withhold the therapy. Equally, where treatment becomes the focus for the expression of the child's more general resentment, insecure parents may seek to end it, being unwilling to accept and cope with their child's hostility. As a result, in many families, treatment may evoke very mixed emotions and some ambivalence, being regarded as a double-edged sword—both useful and distressing.

Treatment procedures required by study children

In this respect, parents of cystic children are especially disadvantaged for most of them are required to give the child a very hefty prophylactic treatment regime. In the families studied, the number of different therapies required each day by the child ranged from one to six, the average being three. Some of these therapies were both time-consuming and complex; for example, all cystic children take replacement pancreatic enzymes with their meals to aid digestion. These can come in capsule form, and many children require them to be opened and sprinkled either on food or in a liquid which they drink. Children vary in the number of capsules they require, the maximum I encountered being 39 a day, 13 with each meal. Clearly, it is an exacting task to open the capsules, mix the enzymes, and get the child to consume the contents.

Most cystic children also require extra vitamins to facilitate growth, and antibiotics to counteract lung infection. These may be relatively easy to administer, normally coming straight from a bottle. Nevertheless, they require a regular routine. Some children need either a special high-protein diet or one free of fats. Chocolate, crisps, chips, and other childish delights may have to be relinquished, accentuating the sick child's sense of being different. In addition, most cystic children require postural drainage and physiotherapy, given either twice or three times daily to clear the lungs. During this, the child must be laid over a special frame or pile of pillows and clapped vigorously in different positions for up to fifteen minutes. Merely keeping the child still and co-operative can be difficult. Finally, some children are advised to sleep in a mist tent to saturate the air which they breathe in at night. Parents are then required to regularly wash down the tent to prevent infection, and to dry out the bedding and pyjamas which become sodden.

Sharing the treatment task

Generally in Northern Ireland it was the mother who assumed the task of giving the child his therapy. This commitment involved her in anything from one to twenty-one extra hours' work a week, variations in time taken being due both to differences in the complexity of the regime required, and also to differences in the mother's own enthusiasm. Usually, the more educated the mother the more time she took to administer treatment, and there were definite social class differences in this respect. Class I and II mothers devoted more time to the task than class III mothers, who in turn spent longer on therapy than class IV or V mothers (Table 16). Similarly, class I and II fathers gave slightly more assistance with treatment than fathers from other socio-economic classes. The only exception to this generalisation was in the case of unemployed fathers who often administered a substantial part of the child's therapy.

Table 16 *Average length of time taken per week by parents in administering the child's treatment, according to sex and social class*

		I and II	III M and III NM	IV and V
Mothers	Time	6 hrs 23 min.	5 hrs 6 min.	4 hrs 55 min.
	No.	14	26	11
Fathers	Time	50 min.	40 min.	46 min.
	No.	11	24	8

Generally, the study mothers seemed perfectly agreeable to this somewhat disproportionate division of labour. Most, being confined to the home, accepted that they were in the best position to shoulder the bulk of the treatment burden. As a result, many had a very positive approach to therapy. To quote a few: 'It's my job. I brought her into the world. No talking will solve it. It's just getting down to it, and getting it done.' 'God gave me that child and it's my job to look after her.' 'I've made up my mind it's a thing I have to do, and that's that.'

However, not all mothers were able to accept the challenge of treatment so positively. A few resented the strain which it imposed on their limited personal resources. Thus one mother of a five-year-old confided:

'I don't blame her for it—on the contrary—but I do resent that I have to do so many things for her, including treatment, and I resent that no one else could do it. I wouldn't trust my husband as much as me.'

Similarly, a few parents of both sexes resented the unremitting nature of the care. Thus one professional father commented:

'I have the feeling that all these strictures make parents neurotic. We couldn't possibly give her physiotherapy twice a day, and therefore we feel very guilty that we don't get up earlier and give it to her. I believe we do what we can. We're not neglecting her. What we're told to do is the ideal—absolute perfection—and we fall short of it and feel guilty.'

In all cases where parents openly admitted to resentment of the treatment task there was evidence of a strained marital relationship.

Similarly in such cases, the actual amount of treatment time was significantly diminished. Thus in five cases where parents were openly at war with each other, the child only received a total of two and a quarter hours' treatment per week from all sources.

In this respect, the findings of this study confirm and elaborate upon those of previous workers (Bozemann *et al.*, 1955; Murstein, 1960). Perhaps nothing reflects family stability and integration so much as the way in which the treatment task is undertaken. Where a father's attitude is less than positive (Henley and Albam, 1955) this can prejudice the mother's ability to cope. Similarly, Bruch and Hewlett (1947), working with diabetic children, found that erratic or poor regulation was often associated with a maternal attitude of self-pity, or a dislike or rejection of the child.

However, in Northern Ireland most parents denied resenting the burden of treatment, although many claimed quite honestly that they disliked it. Most stressed their adaptation to the task; for example, one mother who spent fourteen hours a week on her child said, 'I didn't realise how long I spent until I saw my sister with her child.' Another mother added, 'It just becomes part of your daily routine.' Probably the most widespread feeling was that of a mother who had lost two previous children: 'It's all worthwhile if you can keep him going.'

Treatment help from outside sources

In addition to receiving some assistance from their husbands, many mothers obtained extra help from other sources. Almost half the study children were given occasional therapy by relatives. Nine children received therapy from their siblings, three from a family friend, and eight children who attended a special school for delicate children received physiotherapy and medicaments from staff there.

Generally, the extent of outside help accepted differed according to the mother's need and enthusiasm. Mothers who worked outside the home often substituted the care of relatives and domestics for their own care. For example, baby Anthony, whose mother was a teacher, received six hours' therapy a week from the family housekeeper, three hours' from his mother, and only half an hour on Sunday morning from his father. Robin B., whose father worked away from home, and whose mother became ill, received twice-daily therapy from his fifteen-year-old elder brother.

Children born into the higher socio-economic classes received more additional therapy than children born into class IV and V homes.

Maternal vigilance and sense of responsibility regarding treatment

Mothers differed considerably in their attitude to the assistance they received both from their husband and from other sources. Some were suspicious of it, feeling that others were insufficiently sensitive to the child's ways or lacking in expertise. By contrast, other mothers welcomed assistance; for example, the very stressed mother of one sick and three well children emphasised her dependence on her husband in this respect: 'If it hadn't been for him I would have given up long ago. He's stood by me every time.' And the mother of two cystic children volunteered: 'He would fit in and do half and half. It's not usual for a country father, but it makes a big difference.'

Mothers were quite unequivocal in their attitude to supervision of treatment. Whilst about a third of the study children endeavoured to help themselves with their therapy, only three mothers allowed them to do so without constant personal supervision. Explaining her vigilance in this respect, the mother of an eight-year-old said: 'I feel safer when I've given him everything myself. I know he's definitely had it then.' Similarly, the mother of a nine-year-old commented: 'I always measure it out, and I like to shake the bottle. You can't depend on him that far—you wouldn't know whether it would be mixed right.'

Whilst such vigilance would seem ideal with younger children who might make serious mistakes if left to their own devices, relentless supervision seemed misplaced with older children, many of whom had taken their medicaments for many years and knew exactly what was necessary.

In some extreme cases the mother, through her actions, seemed to be fostering and perpetuating a most unhealthy dependence in her child. Thus one mother, speaking of treatment, said:

'It's become like a religion—a ritual. I think there may come a time when she's older when she'll worry about not being able to get her medicine if I'm not in. She'll want to know who is going to give her her medicine.'

Similarly another mother of a three-year-old found that her daughter would mix her own tablets: 'But she won't take it. I must be there to give her the glass and put it to her mouth. It is only tolerated if I give it to her.'

Fostering dependence of this sort can prejudice the child's development in numerous ways. First, as Schoelly and Fraser (1955) have emphasised when studying families coping with muscular dystrophy, the parent's attention may tend to rivet on treatment to the detriment of the child's wider social and emotional needs. Second, as Bruch and Hewlett (1947) have pointed out in their study of diabetic children, the child thus treated may tend to develop a 'putty-like submissiveness', opting out of the struggle for independence and becoming guilty and discouraged. Treatment may be seen as a symbol of dependence on parents, and during those periods when the child is temporarily stronger, or more anxious, he may resist it.

To some extent, suspicion of others, vigilant supervision of therapy, and the fostering of over-dependence would seem to stem from the same root cause—the mother's pronounced sense of responsibility for the sick child's welfare. Such feelings are obviously exaggerated by the knowledge that the child would fail without therapy. In addition, some mothers may project into the future and envisage their own sense of guilt should anything untoward happen to the child due to lack of care on their part. Thus one mother commented: 'You just have to do it—you can't neglect them. You wouldn't be contented in your mind if you were not doing it. You wouldn't be contented for them or for you.'

Difficulties encountered in giving treatment

Obviously for most present-day families, increasingly unaccustomed to nursing the sick, treatment tasks may pose very real practical difficulties. With the study families, the complexity of the therapeutic regime added to these hardships. Replacement enzymes sometimes 'went off' or were unobtainable. The cost of a high-protein, low-fat diet exceeded some family budgets, and mist tents were noisy, broke down, needed replacement parts and took hours to wash out satisfactorily.

All these difficulties were magnified by the sense of urgency surrounding treatment and the parents' knowledge that somehow, despite obstacles, they must get it done. By contrast to parents of children who receive their therapy from medical personnel, and who can blame such personnel when things go wrong, the parents of cystic children have no one else to share their responsibility; and, as Rosenstein (1970) has emphasised, even slight exacerbations in the disease can produce a 'disproportionate amount of guilt and frustration on their part'. They can therefore be doubly frustrated—by a flare-up in the child's symptoms and by their own inability to control this. This was borne out in the comments of parents, many of whom said that if the child was unwell they felt personally responsible.

Some parents experienced difficulties in giving therapy because of the seemingly unpleasant nature of many treatment procedures and their awareness of the child's own aversion to them. Insecure parents may be especially unwilling to accept responsibility for apparently accentuating the child's pain, either because they cannot bear to see the child suffer, or because, as Lewis (1962) pointed out in his study of acutely ill children in hospital, they cannot tolerate any expression of hostility which such suffering might produce against themselves.

Many parents commented on these points, especially with regard to the physiotherapy. For example, a young professional mother commented of her seven-month-old baby:

> 'He cries invariably, and it makes it more difficult. It's so much better if he doesn't cry for me. Just occasionally he doesn't and then it's terrific. . . . I feel it's a shame that when I get him up the first thing I do is brutalise him.'

Mothers of older children added: 'The hospital will tell you that you're not hurting him—but you seem to be hitting him very hard and that worries us.' Similarly: 'She hated it, she used to screech when she saw the pillows and I felt I was doing more harm than good. It was a sin on her, all that screeching and yelling,' and 'Banging her on her back she doesn't like . . . she's so thin, I always thought it hurted her.'

Such feelings undermined the parent's self-confidence and determination to continue, and were accentuated where the child complained of his treatment. Thus: 'He complains it shakes his tummy and hurts his wound.' 'He doesn't like the position—says you're hurting his head. Makes lots of complaints. Doesn't like sitting so long.' And: 'He hates it. He claims it gives him headaches because of the position. He's never comfortable, says he's very thirsty, has to go to the toilet. He counts every minute. He has no watch but he knows exactly to the minute how long it lasts. That's how much he hates it.'

Occasionally when the protests were sufficiently strenuous, or when the parents were most doubtful of their own abilities, as in the case of some poorly educated class IV and V parents, treatment was actually withheld. Thus the wife of an unskilled labourer who gave her five-year-old daughter little of what was medically recommended said: 'I had trouble with her taking the capsules, but the doctor didn't say I should give them, so I stopped. She wouldn't take them so I never forced her.' Similarly, with the physiotherapy:

> 'I had it explained but she fought a lot with the physiotherapist when she was showing me. The doctor said it would help with her breathing—with her lungs—but she fought so much—she didn't understand it was for her own good, so I didn't bother.'

Another mother, who cheated on the diet, giving her fifteen-year-old fatty foods, said: 'I know in my heart he shouldn't have them—but which is the worst of the two evils?'

Where parents felt it their duty to persist with therapy, even in the face of opposition, they adopted various strategies to effect this. A few endeavoured to minimise the child's sense of difference by pretending such differences didn't exist. Thus the mother of a three-year-old engaged in the following pantomime: 'She looks and wonders why her brother isn't getting a capsule. Sometimes she would say, "Give one to Peter", and I say, "Hurry up Peter—eat up your capsule" so she won't think she's different.'

Other parents faced the problem of obtaining acquiescence more directly. In this respect their behaviours ranged from punitive compulsion to empathetic and sensitive efforts at enlisting voluntary co-operation.

Those parents who met protest head-on with reciprocal force were exemplified by the mother of a two-year-old boy who disliked the replacement enzymes. She commented of his protest: 'If it's too bad, someone holds his two arms and we spoonfeed him.' Similarly, the mother of a six-year-old who was put off capsules by a bad batch said: 'I have to threaten him—take the strap from the box as if to beat him and then he takes it.' Of physiotherapy, the mother of a four-year-old noted: 'He doesn't want to have it done, but I insist, and I have to slap him and make him till I get it done.' Another mother added: 'She fought and cried. The harder she cries, the harder we do it. We reckon it's for her good.'

Bruch and Hewlett (1947), working with diabetic families, noted the damage caused by an attitude of repressive, perfectionistic over-control in families which were able to follow a restricted regime to the letter. Similar damage appeared to be caused by a few study parents who attempted to maintain rigid control over the child's response to therapy by autocratic means. Often such parents showed little sensitivity in other areas of child rearing, being frankly 'slap-happy', and having cowed and depressed children. In fairness, one should say that often such parents were already under strain for reasons other than the child's illness—for example, inadequacy of income or housing, unemployment or an over-large family.

Often in such cases, the child's protests coupled with the parents' sense of stress contributed to an aura of tension in the home; for example, a sixteen-year-old who flatly refused to co-operate with treatment, provoked this comment from his dispirited mother: 'I resent having to nag him, and chase him. It creates a nasty atmosphere in the home.'

Tension was increased where parents disagreed fundamentally about the necessity for treatment. Thus one mother commented on the diet:

'I never give things to his sister in front of him. I say ice
cream's too cold for him, chills his stomach. My husband says,
"Ah, for Heaven's sake, give it to him." He thinks it's awful
keeping it from him. But I think men don't understand.'

While most parents were neither frankly punitive nor overly accepting of protest, a few tried to win their child's co-operation by positive means, making a game of therapy. Thus the mother of a four-year-old only boy said of the physiotherapy and exercises: 'It's more of a game with him. We play Blowing Down the Wolf's House. He really helps himself. He blows and blows and nearly blows you off the settee.' Similarly, the mother of a six-year-old commented: 'I make it into a game. I clapped all his friends' backs. They clapped each other and gave each other injections and clapped Teddy's back.'

Empathetic and positive attitudes of this sort did much to counteract fears, as witnessed by the comments of the mother of a four-year-old who was obliged to sleep in a mist tent: 'I said it was a space ship he was going into, and he used to play in it and switch it on himself. When the man took it away he asked would he bring it back. He thought it was his and a toy.' Similarly, the mother of a three-year-old, who accepted her therapy easily, and reminded her mother whenever she forgot the medicine, said: 'She knows it's going to be done and she lets you. She's very good but sometimes she doesn't feel like it and wriggles around. I make a game of it and play with her and it's quite all right then.'

Occasionally the apparent lack of objective criteria by which to judge the efficacy of treatment leads parents to doubt their own abilities and wonder whether they were administering treatment correctly. This was especially true of the replacement enzymes and physiotherapy. Hence the mother of a four-year-old said: 'I worry about whether I will have to increase it as she grows, and I was never told whether to sprinkle it on the meal or give it before the meal.' Of physiotherapy, a mother said: 'I imagine I'm not doing it right. They only showed me how to do it for 5 minutes;' and: 'I think at the time that I'm not doing it properly, and when I'm not getting anything up I despair of it.'

Frequently, parents failed to appreciate that hospital staff would be glad to explain such procedures in greater detail, or, if they realised this, they were timorous about making contact. During the child's routine reviews they were often too apprehensive, or too anxious to learn about the child's clinical condition to ask questions relating to treatment matters. On such occasions many of them said they forgot what they intended to ask.

Explaining to the child about treatment

Some parents experienced difficulties in explaining the need for treatment to their child. Either they were reticent about explaining too much for fear of frightening the child, or their own basic knowledge concerning the disease was so limited that they were forced to rely on weak generalisations such as, 'It's to make your tummy better.' Whilst explanations of this kind might be sufficient for some younger children, older children frequently found them lacking, especially when faced with continuing symptoms. Thus a nine-year-old whose parents had given therapy 'to make you better' responded that she wouldn't take it any more for she was quite well already. Another girl of the same age, who had been given therapy because 'with a cold you need these to get rid of it', refused treatment saying she no longer had a cold.

As in their attitude to treatment, parents varied considerably in their approach to explaining the illness to the child. Some were very positive, emphasising the preventive aspects. Thus: 'I told her it was to keep her well,' or, 'He must take them to grow.' Generally, this attitude seemed acceptable to the young questioners.

Less acceptable were explanations which emphasised the damaging aspects of the illness in order to effect co-operation. A six-year-old was told, 'It's to get the poison out of your lungs. It sticks in your lungs and it's real bad, full of germs, it gives you pneumonia.' Similarly, an eight-year-old was told her lungs would be damaged if she didn't have it.

Occasionally explanations seemed in danger of creating or feeding frightening fantasies in the children; for example, a four-year-old was told: 'There's a wee mouse down in your chest and you have to get it up.' A six-year-old believed that the physiotherapy was necessary 'to get the yellow stuff out of my chest or it'll go bad'. The parents who offered these explanations seemed surprised that such warnings did little to reduce the child's fears; for example, the mother of a four-year-old said:

'She doesn't like postural drainage at all—even now. She cries whenever you put her down. I explained it to her. I told her if we didn't do it phlegm would be stuck in her and she wouldn't be able to cough it up—but this didn't make any difference at all.'

Some parents found it extremely difficult to be honest in answering their children's questions. Occasionally questions could be very direct, challenging the parents' shaky defences. Thus parents of younger children were asked why only the child had to have the treatment, why other people didn't have it, what part of the body it affected and what it was intended to do. Older children frequently asked how long it would have to continue, and whether they would always need it. At all ages, unbidden fears of death emerged. Thus the mother of a three-year-old said about replacement enzymes: 'I just told him if he takes it it will help him to digest his food. He said, "If I don't take it will I die?" to which I replied, "I don't say you'll die, but I say it'll make you better."' Similarly, the mother of a six-year-old girl explained the enzymes by saying, 'If she doesn't take them she'll be very ill and land herself in hospital. She has to take them in order to live. She said, "Sure I won't die?" and I said, "No, we're talking of living."'

Trusting one's own judgment

Whilst the majority of mothers felt that they could trust their own judgment with regard to treatment, 22 per cent said they could not. Generally these mothers had children who were only recently diagnosed, and consequently they were still endeavouring to master the therapeutic regime. Mothers with greater treatment experience generally felt more secure, for: 'You can think it out for yourself. You learn something more every day,' and 'You sort of get to know.'

Denial of illness and wish to withhold treatment

As mentioned previously (see above, p. 42), approximately one third of the parents continued to deny the severity of their child's disease for many years following diagnosis. Denial was facilitated when the child was well and exhibiting no obvious illness symptoms. At such times many parents—31 per cent of mothers and 37 per cent of fathers—felt an urge to withhold treatment to see whether the child could do without it. Many admitted to actually withholding some of the therapy and watching to see what happened. When the child's symptoms recurred, treatment was recommenced. In addition, a few parents subjected their children to folk medicines, supposed locally to be efficacious. These were given on the assumption that 'We might find a cure. There are times when there is a fantasy that there might be something far removed from medical life—it's a thought that comes into your head.'

Occasionally the child's orthodox treatment was withheld whilst a 'cure' was tried, only to be reinstated when symptoms recurred or the 'cure' was used up. Perhaps such endeavours gave parents additional hope, or diminished their sense of helplessness in the situation.

The child's response to treatment

Just as parents vary considerably in their willingness to explain and pursue therapy, so also children vary in their reactions to it. At one end of the continuum there are those who respond positively and bravely to whatever is required of them. Thus the mother of a four-year-old described him as 'So good about it I think God will get him a cure', and another child of the same age was described as being able to 'take anything—even poison from a spoon'. Cases were cited of children reminding parents to give medicines or do the physiotherapy. One three-year-old was said 'never to forget. He might even take it too often'. A few children appeared almost hypochondriacal. Thus the mother of a six-year-old said: 'She's become very, very fussy.' In these cases the child appeared to mirror the adults' marked concern for his safety and had become absorbed with his own body, anxiously scrutinising his own diet, refusing forbidden food, consuming medicine compulsively, and rigorously guarding himself against draughts and damp. His normal youthful exuberance seemed lost in the process, and, as with the dystrophic children studied by Sherwin and McCully (1961) or the cardiac children observed by Bergmann (1965) normal age-appropriate strivings for independence seemed diminished as a consequence.

At the other end of the continuum, there were children who refused treatment consistently and, in a few extreme cases, absolutely abandoned it. As one mother said: 'He kicks and fights against it continuously. It's an exhausting battle.'

Occasionally, hostility was provoked by the apparently punitive nature of the treatment—the swallowing of unpleasant substances, the limitations of good intake, or the need for immobilisation. Punitive fantasies were accentuated by the lack of privacy and loss of independence occasioned by the illness. Often protest was out of all proportion to the severity of the treatment regime, even minimal stresses being reacted to with unnecessary violence. This was especially true where additional impositions were added to the usual burden. As with the orthopaedic cases studied by Bergmann (1965), and the children with malignant diseases observed by Green (1967), cystic children often responded excessively to changes in school, family moves, discord between parents or the death of relatives or friends. The parents were perpetually reminded of the need for constancy: 'You have to keep your promise with him—everything has to be exact.'

Often the child realised that treatment protests were unacceptable to parents, and for fear of prejudicing vital support (Chodoff et al., 1964) he endeavoured to choke down his natural hostility and comply. The child's response to treatment varied then according to his mood. One day he might accept it easily, another day refuse. Thus the mother of a six-year-old described physiotherapy as: 'easy depending on the mood he's in. If he's in a good mood he goes and gets down on the floor. If he's in a bad mood we have to force it on him.' Another boy who was on a strict diet was said to demand chocolate only when 'he was in a nasty mood'.

Treatment protest could be used as a means of expressing the child's more general dissatisfaction with being ill, perhaps being of actual value to the child by affording him some outward trapping on which to attach more pervasive and less acceptable fears. Thus regular treatment, accompanied by regular protest, gave him some controlled way of expressing his apprehensions, and in all probability, because of his parents' sensitivity, a good means of arresting support and attention. Similarly treatment protest behaviour could be used by the child as a means of expressing more general dissatisfaction with domestic affairs. Thus the birth of a new brother or sister, and consequent jealousy, often produced a refusal to co-operate, presumably in the hope of securing extra cosseting.

Even from earliest days, children seemed extremely efficient in assessing accurately the strength of their parents' convictions with regard to the necessity for treatment. Thus the mother of a ten-year-old, speaking of his pre-school days, said: 'I couldn't get over how cunning he became with treatments—watching me for my reactions.' The mother of a six-year-old said: 'When she knows you mean it, she'll take it.' The mother of a five-year-old who took 'his cocktail' of three medicines mixed up together four times a day, said: 'He takes it very well, no complaints, no refusals, *no option!*'

This ability to interpret parental decisiveness correctly meant that parents who wished to be vigilant about therapy had to maintain an unremittingly positive approach to it. None the less, some children certainly attempted to manipulate their parents—both generally and in order to avoid therapy—by accentuating their own misery. A six-year-old girl was said to be: 'Very, very shrewd. She could play on it. She would say, "You can't hit me because I'm not strong".' When her mother replied that she could, and would, hit her if she didn't co-operate the child rejoined, 'Then I'll write to my doctor and he'll barge you!' Similarly, a father who felt he was hurting his seven-year-old son when giving therapy found 'he would play on it, and say, "Don't do it. You're hurting me."'

Generally, children seemed best able to accept therapy without excessive upset where it became part of a well-established and unavoidable routine. This was especially true for children who had no real experience of an alternative existence, thus pre-school children, who were placed on treatment as infants, seemed to accept their lot with most ease. Similarly, only children were at an advantage.

As soon as the child became fully conscious of the difference between himself and other people, he was more likely to question what was happening. Going to school had, in many instances, a significant effect on the child's response to therapy. Capsules became a source of embarrassment and were thrown away or taken furtively in the cloakroom. Many children refused physiotherapy when their friends were around, saying it was 'a waste of time', something that hurt, or that it occasioned undue subtle fears; for instance, a ten-year-old commented: 'Sometimes I get worried if I don't feel better when the draining's finished. Sometimes I feel better before I do it, and worse afterwards.'

At this stage the importance of parental attitude was most apparent. Where the parents accepted the illness manifestations without shame or evasion, and where they supported the child and emphasised the preventive nature of therapy, the child himself seemed best able to accept it. The converse was also true—lies, evasions, or plain denial on the part of the parents often produced near panic reactions in the child. Thus a ten-year-old boy who had been told nothing about his illness by his parents began 'to rebel against his treatment, even though he should be getting it'. Eventually he refused every form of medicine and physiotherapy and declined to visit either the doctor or the dentist. His mother said: 'He realised there is something wrong with him and he doesn't like to be different, and you try and talk to him and he won't listen.' In actual fact, when illness was mentioned, this boy normally got up and ran away. Although the mother had studiously avoided the subject for many years, the child had recently asked why he had to take medicine, and why no one else had to take it. His mother replied, 'Because you were born with a little bit missing from the parts to digest your food.' This prompted the question, 'Will I always have to take it? Can't I stop taking it when I'm thirteen, when I'm a teenager?' to which the mother said she didn't know, only doctors could tell. This poor mother, who was herself embarrassed by the whole subject of illness, was married to a totally denying husband. She commented, 'I didn't dare tell my husband I'd told him. He would have been so cross. This is a terrible thing to tell a child. Do you tell this to a child? I don't know at all.'

Other children refused treatment because of the frightening fantasies which they had woven concerning it; for example, an eight-year-old girl refused to enter a mist tent, 'She thought it was a cellophane bag and I had her scared of them and she just sat in the tent and shook and she was terrified. "I'm going to die. I'm going to die," she said.'

Just as some parents withhold treatment in their attempts to deny the severity of the child's illness, so also some children refuse treatment in the hope of denying the reality of their condition. This was especially true of older children for whom the illness had become a social embarrassment. They hoped that by forgoing their medicaments the symptoms would also disappear magically. In this respect my findings are in agreement with those of Lawler *et al.* (1966) and also with those of Chodoff (1959), who cited instances in which children with muscular dystrophy repudiated their wheelchairs in the hope that the disease would also disappear.

Differences in the actual nature of the treatments produced differences in response. Table 17 indicates that the therapy most disliked was postural drainage and physiotherapy. Children of all

Table 17 *Type of therapy and degrees of child protest and parental dislike occasioned by it (n = 58)*

Type of therapy	Children receiving therapy (%)	Children receiving therapy who protested against it (%)	Parents administering therapy who disliked giving it (%)
Replacement enzymes	100	43	22
Antibiotics and vitamins	86	14	3
Physiotherapy and postural drainage	82	77	51
Mist tent	31	38	36
Diet	27	18	30

ages disliked this because it limited their freedom and interrupted their play. Also, whilst physiotherapy was in progress, feelings of anger and frustration could not be discharged normally by moving around. They were therefore pent up and seeking expression. In addition, the very obviousness of physiotherapy meant that it could not be got over quickly and furtively but was a constant reminder to the child of his frailty. In the same way, replacement enzymes were disliked by 43 per cent of children not only because of their strong taste, but because of their obviousness which produced questioning and general embarrassment in social situations. By contrast, changes in diet and antibiotics, which were relatively unobtrusive and more usual, were disliked by very few.

In all these respects there was a close relationship between the attitudes of both parents and children, and undoubtedly the attitudes of one modified and altered the attitudes of the other.

A further factor to be considered in terms of the child's reaction to his treatment was the actual survival value it had for him. Generally, less well children responded best to therapy. This was substantiated by the parents' comments. Thus the mother of an eight-year-old said: 'When she's not well she would take anything to make her feel better.' A five-year-old who normally refused physiotherapy would get the pillows and get up on them when she was sick. As her mother said: 'She knows in her own mind more than we give her credit for.' A sixteen-year-old who refused every other form of therapy accepted physiotherapy from his mother because 'He feels that's keeping his other lung all right. That will keep him alive all right. That's on his mind.'

Finally, one should mention the considerable benefit in terms of the child's response to treatment which accrued from proper supportive parental explanations. Where the child was aware that the parents had his best interests at heart, and only gave treatment to potentiate his health and ease his suffering, treatment protests were less severe. The mother of a seven-year-old girl demonstrated this point. Previously the child had been persistently questioning the reason for, and protesting against, treatment; so the mother, observing her at doll play, said casually: 'If you have a little girl when you grow up, and that little girl isn't well, and her doctor says she must have exercises and medicine or she'll get sick, will you say to yourself, "Poor wee thing, I won't bother. I'll just leave her peacefully," or will you say, "Oh, goodness me. I must do my best to keep her well so she can grow up to be a mummy herself"?' The little girl sat and thought, and eventually said: 'I'll give her the medicines and help her grow up.' 'Well, that's what I'm doing for you,' said the mother. Splendidly the treatment protests vanished.

Where the child is properly informed and supported in this way, treatment can afford him a chance to grow emotionally, through learning to master his anxiety and hostility. Equally the intimacy of the contacts necessitated by the need to administer treatments may help him to develop richer and more meaningful relationships with his parents than might otherwise be possible.

7

The child in hospital

'It pulled my flesh asunder, like parting with part of myself.'
(*Mother of an infant, taken into hospital*)
'When he went in it used to be me who was crying and Sister
would say she didn't know who to put in the cot—me or the boy.'
(*Mother of a six-year-old*)
'I didn't like hospital because I was away from home and
Mummy was crying for me—she told me.'
(*Seven-year-old*)

It is now well recognised that the unsupported hospitalisation of a
child—especially a very young child—can have profound effects on
his physical and emotional growth. Encompassing, as it does,
crippling feelings of inadequacy, strangeness and loneliness,
hospitalisation can produce actual physical wasting and deteriora-
tion, accentuate pain, and prejudice both immediate and long-term
personality growth. Emotional disturbance is reflected both in the
child's behaviour on the ward and also by adverse reactions on his
return home (Jessner and Kaplan, 1948; Robertson, 1952; Jackson
et al., 1952; Jackson *et al.,* 1953; Schaffer and Callender, 1959).

The root cause of such disturbance would seem to be the removal
of the young child—all those under three and most of those under
five—from the mother upon whom he depends for emotional and
social support. Providing better play and educational facilities, an
accepting ward environment or mother substitutes in the form of

good and devoted nurses may lessen the anguish of older children but does little to console these younger children for the loss of their mother (Prugh *et al.*, 1953; Illingworth and Holt, 1955; Vaughan, 1957; Plank *et al.*, 1959). Indeed, many younger children will not accept substitute mothers, their sense of abandonment being heightened by any usurpation of maternal comforting (Bergmann, 1965; Bowlly, 1971). For this reason many paediatricians now advocate either the child's attendance on an outpatient basis (Knudson and Natterson, 1960), a programme of parental participation in hospital nursing care (Spence, 1947; Bierman, 1956) or the establishment of a mother and child unit (Spence, 1946, 1947, 1951; MacCarthy 1957; MacCarthy *et al.*, 1962; Craig and McKay, 1958; Riley *et al.*, 1965). Recently, attendance in such a unit has been shown with this younger age group to reduce significantly the emotional and infective complications attendant on minor surgery (Brain and Maclay, 1968).

But loneliness and a sense of isolation and abandonment are not confined solely to the very young child. Older hospitalised children also experience such feelings. Similarly, hospitalisation may threaten their nascent sense of independence. Unlike the adult who chooses hospital treatments for himself, the child is 'taken to the doctors by his parents and has had no control over the process that finally brought him to hospital' (Stacey *et al.*, 1970). Once there he is often turned, without adequate explanation or preparation, from a mobile, assertive child, whose opinions are valued, into a passive recipient of treatment. Not only does such passivity imply loss of identity and status, but it also decreases the child's chances of mastering basic skills, and is therefore resented. Teenagers may become especially disturbed by enforced passivity, viewing restrictions as punishment for some wrong-doing (Easson, 1968). Similarly, immobility may hinder the normal discharge of negative emotions through movement, increasing feelings of frustration and animosity, which may well up when additional and unexpected treatment procedures are imposed on the child. Conversely, enforced passivity may accentuate feelings of apathy and resignation, which can only be counteracted by giving the child some active role in his treatment.

The average hospital ward is still markedly different from most normal homes, and this very difference may confuse and frighten many young children, who do not know how to act in the situation. A new and appropriate role—that of child patient—will have to be learnt, often overnight. This may undermine the young child's self-confidence, making him more apprehensive subsequently in other social situations. Children with less well developed social skills or from more permissive home backgrounds are especially disadvantaged in this respect (Stacey *et al.*, 1970).

The child's actual physical condition will also affect his response to hospitalisation. Very ill children, or children with dramatic and frightening symptoms, will respond very differently from children in better health who go in for less urgent treatment. Pain may evoke feelings of anger and resentment, and because the child may be 'unable to distinguish between feelings of suffering caused by the disease inside the body and suffering imposed on him from the outside for the sake of curing the disease' (Freud, 1952), the child in pain may respond to staff with open antagonism. In turn, such antagonism may accentuate his pain (Easson, 1968). Where pain is long-lasting, the child may respond excessively to even trivial setbacks or changes in routine.

Children of all ages may fear painful treatments, such as injections, and these fears may colour their relationships with the staff who are giving the treatment. In much the same way as some children view home treatment as punishment for wrong-doing, many view hospital procedures as evidence of rejection or an attack on themselves. Fears of mutilation and permanent damage may be accentuated where the child needs surgery (Blom, 1958; Freud, 1952; Miller, 1951; Pearson, 1941). This would seem especially true where anaesthesia is necessary (Levy, 1945). As a result, some children may experience distortions in personality growth, both at the time and for many years to follow. The child may view himself as less adequate, develop a 'heightened anxiety about bodily intactness', and as a consequence feels worthless and dispirited. In addition, possibly for the first time, 'the parents' helplessness, anxiety, and incapacity to protect the child' (Calef, 1959) may become painfully clear, and, at the time when he needs them most, the child may view his parents as failing him. This feeling would seem especially true where the child is seriously ill, and when he begins to sense his parents' very real fears for his survival. In such cases, fears of death may begin to present themselves. Deaths of older children—either on the ward, or known through the outpatient clinic—may accentuate such fears, especially if death is hastily denied and the child is deprived of the opportunity to discuss it adequately. Teenage patients, who do fully comprehend the irreversibility of death, are perhaps the most sensitive in this respect, and death fears may produce a total denial of all that is happening.

Very little objective study has yet been made of the ways in which children tolerate and live with such fears. Langsley (1961) suggests that denial, repression and regression may help. Morrissey (1963) found that, despite severe or noticeable anxiety, 70 per cent of the fifty children he studied made a good overall adjustment to their hospitalisation for leukaemia. The child's previous character structure, the quality of the parent-child relationships and the actual medical circumstances of the child were significant factors in attaining this adjustment. He concluded: 'Two children may have similar levels of anxiety but the anxiety may operate differently in the two individuals; one child may be emotionally paralyzed, and the other use resources constructively to keep anxiety under control.' In this respect, his findings agree with those of Tropauer et al. (1970), who, observing cystic children, concluded: 'It is not the existence of anxiety per se that handicaps the sick child and intensifies his invalidism but rather its degree and his methods of dealing with it.'

But the child patient is not the only one to be worried in the situation. His parents may also fear for his safety. Previous fears for his survival, and personal insecurities engendered by the diagnosis (above, p. 46) may be accentuated, and, in addition, visiting the child in hospital may produce a host of practical difficulties for parents and much emotional stress, not least that occasioned by observance of the child's anguish in a situation in which they feel powerless to help. In turn, parental upset may increase that of the child, who may anxiously question half-hidden tears, or silently and correctly interpret his parents' less obvious emotions. This chapter will therefore deal not only with the difficulties encountered by young chronically sick children in terms of hospitalisation, but also with those of older children and their parents. The reactions of one to the situation will be seen to influence or accentuate those of the other.

All but one of the fifty-eight study children had been hospitalised at some stage. On average, the children had been taken in for diagnostic testing or emergency treatment four times prior to the survey, which took place when the average age of the group was five years. The length of time spent in hospital varied considerably, one eight-year-old spending only one week there, another sixteen-year-old sustaining at least sixty-three admissions and spending at least 192 weeks as an inpatient.

Hospitalisation of the young child

As might be predicted from the previous discussion, 61 per cent of young cystic children exhibited some signs of emotional distress whilst hospitalised. The most usual responses were excessive crying and an attempt to cling tenaciously to the mother. Occasionally, such protest behaviour was superseded by despair, the child lying listless and apparently uncaring in his cot. More rarely, the child appeared to withdraw from the mother, or became violently angry with her when she visited (Table 18 gives the incidence of these behaviours, as reported by the mothers).

Behaviours indicative of emotional distress were seen from earliest days; for example, the mother of a five-month-old baby said: 'Every time I went in she was screeching. Once I nursed her she was all right.' Another boy of the same age cried so excessively that his mother began to cry in sympathy, with the consequence that her distressed husband forbade her to return.

Table 18 *Behaviours indicative of emotional distress in young hospitalised cystic children, as reported by their mothers* (%)

Cried excessively	41
Clung to mother	41
Became passive and listless	18
Became angry with mother	13
Sucked his thumb	13
Withdrew from mother	11
Refused to speak to mother	11
Became angry with sibs	7·5
Rocked, or banged head	7·5
No.	57

The mother of an eleven-month-old found: 'She lay still and passive. She only cried when the nurse came up. She knew when the nurse came for injections, she knew and she cried. She hit the nurse when she gave her medicines. She looked at me as if looking for help.' The mother of a sixteen-month-old boy found that he cried excessively and clung to her during visiting hours. She reported: 'He doesn't like white coats now, he cries when he sees them, and he doesn't like stethoscopes. He cries when he sees those too.'

Most mothers correctly interpreted these behaviours as indicative of a need on the tiny child's part for constancy and reassurance; for example, the mother of a baby girl said: 'She was clingy because she was so ill. She found she needed me so. I was the person who could understand her—she needed me.'

Slightly older children seemed confused by the change in environment. For example, a girl of twenty months was taken in for two weeks' routine testing. Her mother said: 'She was so cross and so confused, she cried so much and kept calling for her nanny.'

Changes in the child's physical wellbeing or actual wasting consequent on hospitalisation were also noticeable; thus an eighteen-month-old, in for routine testing, became 'very limp, very tearful, funny at times, limp, not full of life as usual.' A four-year-old experienced a 'shock to her system'. Her mother commented: 'She did pine away. She was crying when I left her but the flesh walked off her in three weeks. If I'd been able to stay with her I would have.' Another four-year-old girl was sick and failed to thrive in hospital. 'She fretted a terrible lot and neither put on weight nor looked well during those seven weeks, but when I got her home she put on weight and grew.'

Those mothers whose children responded with aggression were most especially distressed. Three years after the event, one mother cried whilst describing to me how her three-year-old had withdrawn from her whilst hospitalised. 'She just refused to speak to me. When she was walking again she wouldn't look near me, she didn't want me. I was really rejected, you know.' The mother of a four-year-old boy who needed constant hospitalisation blamed his hostility towards her on the fact that it was she who had to take him into hospital. By contrast, her husband, who was still favoured by the child, normally went to collect him on discharge day. Because of distance and the presence of younger children at home this mother couldn't get up to visit him often

'and then he would take a spite against me sort of a way and get on against me. He threw the toys I brought away down the corridor, and he was at me that bad I couldn't talk to him. I had to turn the other way, away from him to let him see how much he hurt me. When I did speak he said, "Don't talk to me." Sister sent me home, she thought it wasn't doing him much good. He was awful cold when I was visiting and she thought it was shock.'

Not all mothers who were met by aggression were so restrained. Some met force with force; for example, the mother of a three-year-old hit him soundly when he hit her in the face and smashed her glasses on the floor.

Sadly, those mothers who were subjected to aggression upon visiting seemed to have markedly strained relationships with their children subsequently. Whether this resulted from the experience, or whether both were produced by some pre-existing disturbance in relationship I cannot tell. In several cases the difficulties were so great as to require the intervention of the father, both to maintain peace between the protagonists and also to supervise and administer home-based therapy.

Occasionally hospital staff endeavoured to break the child of some 'undesirable' habit whilst he was in their charge. Whilst this did not appear to happen often, and certainly not in the most enlightened establishments, where it occurred it caused additional pain to both mother and child. For instance, a child who was very attached to her dummy 'squealed and squealed' after it was removed. A girl of twenty months who was used to a bottle morning and night 'cried an awful lot' when deprived of it. A three-year-old who normally slept in a nappy 'was so scared in case she wet the bed that she couldn't sleep properly in hospital when it was removed'. Parents of such children noted their pain and felt useless, being unable to intervene.

Perhaps the greatest source of anguish for young children was the non-appearance of the needed mother. In this respect, I was distressed to find that 44 per cent of the study children were not visited daily in hospital by their parents. Four children had never been visited at all, and a further fourteen children were visited at best twice a week (Table 19 gives details of the average number of parental visits per week, as reported by the mother).[1]

Non-visiting mothers rationalised their absence in various ways; for example, the mother of an eighteen-month-old said: 'He was

---

[1] In this context, it was interesting to find that socio-economic factors seemed of little significance in determining the extent of parental visiting. Mothers in classes I and II visited, on average, 5·1 times a week, mothers from class III visited 4·9 times a week and mothers from classes IV and V 5·0 times a week.

only in for a week. I didn't bother to visit. It just upsets him, and it gives them more trouble to nurse.' Another mother who had lost one child couldn't bear to visit in case the second child also died.

Two mothers said they were persuaded not to visit by the nursing staff. In all four cases, the children were markedly anxious and distressed both at the time and for years to follow. One mother who had left her twelve-month-old daughter alone for a week said:

Table 19 *Average number of parental hospital visits per week, as reported by the mother*

'Never	4
Once	7
Twice	7
Three times	4
Four times	2
Five times	1
Every day	32
No.	58

'It nearly killed her—emotionally and physically both. It was one of those terrible things. Rather than have the child crying, I wouldn't go and visit her. I should have gone and stayed with her. It was crazy, my mistake for not being with her. She used to wake up and scream and scream, and that went on for five or six years. I do honestly think it stemmed from those days in hospital. They said she cried all the time. It was such an awful mistake to have made—but that was nine years ago. I was crazy. They took her from me and she screamed and screamed and I did nothing. Now I would realise this wasn't on, but things were done differently then.'

The mother of a two-year-old boy reported:

'In that hospital they said the best thing was not to go and see him, and I didn't go for three days. When I did I never forgot it—he put his arms out and clung. I couldn't even put him down in his cot. He seemed to think he was left in there and would never see us again. He was like a wee ghost. They thought if we didn't go near he'd forget us, and Sister didn't seem to want us, but my husband said to stay anyway—it was for his good. After that I decided to work him at home myself.'

Parents who visited rarely—at best once or twice a week—often cited distance as the reason for their absence. Many of them lived in excess of forty miles from the child's hospital and, in the absence of adequate public transport, had to wait for the weekend to be driven there by relatives. Generally, such parents were very concerned for the hospitalised child, fearing he would fret, but feeling themselves unable to do much about it. Communication also posed a problem. As one country mother put it: 'Being so far away, and knowing he was so far away, and not being able to visit was very upsetting. You don't get much satisfaction on the 'phone—just "he's all right".'

Even where parents managed to visit regularly, their problems—and those of the child—were very far from solved. Whilst parents might be welcomed with joy when they arrived, when it was time for departure 'the heavens opened' if the child wasn't already asleep. Watching the child's suffering, and being unable to assuage it, accentuated the parents' pain. Often, in desperation, mothers resorted to tricks or lies in the hope of averting the anticipated distress. Thus the mother of a two-year-old commented: 'I used to have to shoot out quick before he saw me go, which was upsetting. I don't like leaving him.' A mother who found her child much quieter after hospital said: 'I used to try and slip out whilst she wasn't looking—but then she got fly and would hold on to me—then I just had to walk out of the room.' Another mother added, 'I had to get away by telling lies. I sat there all day and played games, and then I said, "I have to go home and make dinner. I'll be back up later," but I never went back up.' Many parents appreciated that these strategies undermined their bond with the child, and this also distressed them.

Similarly, the mother's overall stress was accentuated when she was forced to choose between being with her sick child or remaining at home with his well brothers and sisters. Whatever choice was made, inevitably she felt neglectful. In this context, some mothers said how grateful they would be if hospital visiting arrangements were altered so that grandparents or close relatives could also take a turn. This need seemed especially urgent when the child was largely reared by the grandparent and the loss of this beloved figure was of equal significance to the loss of a parent.

A few mothers felt that, by handing the child's care over to the nurses, they were failing in their own maternal duties; for instance, the mother of a two-year-old commented: 'I didn't like to see him going in—I had the feeling I wanted to work with him myself. It's foolish, I know—but just the nature of mothers.' Resentment thus formed occasionally expressed itself in the mother's negative behaviour towards nursing staff, or in her comments concerning them. Thus one very anxious mother commented: 'The majority of nurses—not the doctors—try to make you feel inferior and dependent on them. They make you feel small. Doctors never make you feel small—they welcome you and make you feel accepted.'

Where a parent was able to live in with the sick child and assume responsibility for his care, personality problems seemed minimised, and many parents spoke warmly of the facilities that had been afforded to them in mother-child units. In one case, to facilitate rooming in by the mother of two cystic children, whenever one was taken ill both were admitted simultaneously, thereby keeping all the family together. Comments such as 'it was great. They left us alone and we played together' were frequent. Days spent together in this way generally had a very positive effect on the relationship of the parent and child, and consequent feelings of closeness were accentuated. As one mother said, who spent four weeks in with her eleven-month-old child: 'That time brought me very close to her. She shows her love more now.' Occasionally bonding thus engendered became exaggerated and had less positive repercussions in terms of the child's other relationships. Thus several children were described as not wanting their fathers when they returned home: 'She just looked at me. That annoyed my husband—but I can't help it.' 'She couldn't abide anyone else near her, not her grandfather or her brothers, only me.'

Constant visiting could be advantageous for parents in other respects not least being the diminution of pre-existing fears. Often, when the child was hospitalised, fears for his survival, which might have been dormant since diagnosis, were re-activated. This was especially true where the child was admitted to the same hospital or even the same ward as that in which a previous sibling had died. Then it became imperative for the parent to ascertain his safety: 'I had to go no matter what it cost. I had to go—even if he was lying sleeping. Then I came back satisfied.'

Some parents found that as a result of their hospital experiences they were better able to accept the facts of their own child's illness. Thus the mother of a five-year-old commented: 'It was a good thing seeing her in hospital—for there were so many worse cases and we were quite glad to have her with cf. It had a therapeutic effect.'

Practical problems occasioned for parents by visiting

Balanced against these positive effects there were practical problems —some of awesome proportions—occasioned by visiting. In a few instances parents travelled 180 miles a day to be with their child in hospital. One mother spent the family's entire savings of £250 in taking the child to a London teaching hospital for two months' diagnostic testing. Eventually she ran out of money and had to sleep in a welfare hostel. In some families, visiting costs consumed over a quarter of the family's weekly income, producing deprivations in terms of food and comfort. These difficulties existed for some parents despite the child's age, but were especially pressing when the parents felt the child needed them emotionally and practically.

Behaviour difficulties exhibited by young children upon return home from hospital

Eighty per cent of the young children in this study exhibited some difficulties in settling back into their home environment following hospitalisation. The most usual difficulty was extra-demanding behaviour, the child endeavouring in different ways to attract his parents' attention. Forty-two per cent of children behaved in this way. Often the child clung physically to the mother, refusing to allow her out of his sight. Thus the mother of a two-year-old 'couldn't go upstairs without his being with me. He followed me everywhere.' The mother of a three-year-old said: 'I couldn't leave him to go into the kitchen without his screaming at me.' Most mothers correctly interpreted this behaviour as resulting from the young child's fear of further abandonment; for instance, the mother of a four year old said: 'He wouldn't have anything to do with the other children. He wouldn't leave me. He would scream at everyone. I can understand it. He thought I was going to leave him again.' Similarly, 'he was always watchful, worried in case you would leave him again.'

Generally, mothers could accept this form of attention-seeking behaviour and most responded to it with additional affection: 'We coaxed her round as nice as possible. We didn't like her to be too cross.' 'I put her on my knee and nursed her. I let other things go, and read to her. We sat by the fire and read.'

More difficult to cope with were the aggressive behaviours exhibited by some children, especially those who were rarely or never visited; for instance, one boy whose mother described hospital as 'a holiday camp' and never bothered to visit her son because 'he was always having a great time there' found that on return 'he got very wicked with his little sister. He would scrab her face a lot and hit her and throw cups around.' Another mother whose infrequent hospital appearances were due to poverty and the presence of younger children in the home, found her four-year-old son 'very, very cross. Angry. You have to force him to do everything.' Ultimately her relationship with the child was undermined to the extent that 'He works a lot better for his father, for his father seems to be doing something for his benefit, whereas he thinks I'm brow-beating him.'

Occasionally, as with hostility exhibited on the ward, the child's aggression following hospital was countered by parental force; for example: 'I did what he wanted at first, but then his demands became too much. He became very cheeky and in the end I had to check him,' and 'You just have to be firm with them and say "no". If you don't, the children would play you up terribly.'

Other more subtle difficulties following hospitalisation often presented a greater challenge to parental skills. Sleep difficulties were most pressing. The mother of a two-year-old said, 'You couldn't get her to go to sleep. She screamed and you couldn't get her to settle.' A baby of nine months, who was hospitalised for six weeks 'was used to the light in hospital. When she woke up here afterwards she woke up screaming.' The mother of a baby girl, hospitalised from two to eight months of age, said: 'Afterwards she didn't know me. She just cried for the nurses. I used to feed her from behind so she didn't see my face.' Another mother found that her eighteen-month-old daughter 'being used to the cot in hospital, tended to stay in the cot for ages—she just lay in it—seemed to think that was where she should stay.'

Difficulties of this nature not only distressed the parents by reminding them of the child's previous anguish, but also accentuated the practical and emotional problems they themselves experienced in dealing with the sick child. Over-dependency on the mother, exaggerated by fears of abandonment produced by hospitalisation, occasionally produced resentment on the part of the father, which militated against the mother's ability to give treatment. Similarly, long-term rivalry between brothers and sisters was often triggered off by the young child's excessive demands following unsettling hospital experiences and his parents' well-meaning attempts to alleviate these.

Finally, additional stresses were produced for parents where the child's hospital experiences had an aversive effect on his subsequent relationships with medical staff. For instance, the mother of a three-year-old became 'upset, especially if I had to take him back to hospital for X-rays. He would shout and scream. It was very upsetting.' Frequently, anticipation of such difficulties contributed to the parents' failure to adequately prepare the child for subsequent testing or hospitalisation. Thus even on occasions when they knew the child was likely to be kept in, some assured him of the reverse, unwittingly contributing to his ultimate insecurity.

Hospitalisation of the school-age child

Generally, older children fared better in hospital, being more socially competent, better able to withstand separation, and more adept at containing their anxieties. Parents acknowledged such changes with relief; for instance, the mother of a ten-year-old commented:

'He is a very, very good patient. In fact, he enjoys the social life. He takes the biscuits round and the time he was in with the croup he fell in love with a blonde girl and when he went up for check-ups he would say, "I wonder will Evie be there?" He still talks about people he met in hospital when he was five. He has a great personality, he's a great entertainer. We would go to visit him and he would entertain us. He's not in the least in awe of doctors and nurses. He treats them as an equal.'

Similarly, the mother of a six-year-old who spent three weeks as an in-patient, said:

'He settled down very well and loved hospital, so we didn't have to worry. The treatment he was having wasn't painful and he enjoyed it, and the first night he was home he was crying and said he missed the nurses. He was the youngest in the ward and the older boys were good to him.'

Problems seemed lessened by the fact that school-age children could talk about their experiences, both while they were happening and afterwards. Also, parents felt better able to prepare older children for hospital visits. Although many in-patient visits were of an emergency nature, none the less, they could be discussed—albeit briefly—beforehand, and occasionally, where time permitted, older children even experienced 'great fun packing their own things'.

In addition, older children were better able to appreciate the value of hospital treatment, and some were thought by their parents to view hospital more positively because it had become associated for them with real physical improvement; for instance, the mother of a six-year-old boy commented:

'Before that he had no energy. He wouldn't go out and play.
He used to sit round the house all the time. I used to try and
chase him out to get some fresh air. After hospital, he was
more robust and wanted to play rough games. He wanted to
play football and things like that.'

As with home-based treatment, a positive attitude to hospital was occasionally fostered in older, more seriously ill children by the fact that they were fully able to appreciate the value of all that was being done for them by hospital staff. As one mother put it: 'He knows when he's sick and there are no complaints at all. Usually he's that sick he doesn't care.'

Occasionally, as with younger children, such positive effects were jeopardised by well-meaning but over-enthusiastic attempts at breaking the child's 'unacceptable' habits. For example, a fourteen-year-old who had previously accepted hospital uncomplainingly announced one day that 'he didn't like hospital'. His mother added: 'On a cold day he just got his coat on, and walked out. They were trying to get him off the smoking, and one doctor caught him in the toilet, and so he just marched out, and they caught him down the main road.'

In a few cases traumatic early experiences associated with painful procedures such as injections and drips, produced long-lasting fears of hospital, which generalised even to the outpatient clinic. Thus, whilst the majority of children seemed to enjoy their regular check-ups, getting extra attention, little treats and jokes when they went to the clinic, a few were so afraid of being 'kept in' that they made themselves ill prior to clinic visits.

In my conversations with twenty-eight school-age cystic children, 47 per cent expressed a fear of going into hospital, 50 per cent of being ill, and 65 per cent of being hurt. Usually these fears merged. Whilst the child said he was afraid of hospital, he was actually afraid of fantasies associated with weakness or painful procedures; for example, a six-year-old boy who claimed erroneously to have been in 'a hundred days the last time' said he hated hospital because 'they had a needle. I don't like needles because they make you bleed. I don't like bleeding because you bleed to death. That could happen to me because it's sore.' Similarly, another boy of the same age was frightened of hospital because 'when the doctor came I was worried in case she would do something frightening that would hurt'. An eight-year-old said, 'They took my stitches out. They put me in a bed and tucked me up. I thought they'd got a big knife and I started to scream.' A fourteen-year-old became afraid when 'they put a buzzing thing on my back and put bandages round it and turned it up so high in volume. I didn't know what was going on. I thought I was going to be electrocuted.'

Simple explanations concerning the reason for, and nature of, these procedures would have done much to contain and allay the frightening fantasies, and this fact was accepted by virtually all the children I spoke to. For instance, an eight-year-old girl stated: 'If I'd been told, it would have helped. It would have made me feel not as frightened as I would be.' A boy of seven commented: 'I was frightened when I was X-rayed. I thought I was going to get an operation. It would have helped if the doctor had told me.' Similarly, fears concerning actual procedures and the child's lack of control over these might have been counteracted by giving the child some means of alerting staff to his needs when they became pressing. For example, children immobilized for a drip, or tests of stomach contents, would have welcomed a buzzer on their bed to press when they became afraid and wanted reassurance. One ten-year-old boy hated it when, unsedated, 'they put tubes down my nose to my stomach to get juice. I couldn't talk or eat or anything. I couldn't blow my nose. One time I vomited and I thought I'd choke myself.' A buzzer would have brought immediate aid and greatly supplemented this boy's own very considerable fortitude. Despite his anxieties, this boy was able to console his weeping mother when she visited. He indicated that she should go home because she was crying so much, and later when he could talk again said he hadn't wanted her 'to ruin her eye make-up'.

Although I did not specifically ask about this, many mothers voluntarily confided that their children had become more aware and afraid of dying as a result of hospital experiences (Burton, 1973b). For example, the mother of an eight-year-old said: 'They talked about her, at the bottom of the bed. She told me. They said that she wasn't going to do. She said, "Don't leave me Mummy. Don't go away whilst it happens."' In some cases such thoughts could have been prevented if medical and nursing staff had followed the essential rule of never discussing even the youngest patient within his hearing. In other instances, the possibility of impending death seemed to emerge unbidden, the child himself making the necessary logical extrapolation. Then, if such thoughts were voiced, he was often looking for reassurance and comfort.

While most school-age children were able to assess the need for hospitalisation objectively and did not therefore view it as an abandonment on the part of their parents, several none the less felt jealous of those who remained at home: 'I get jealous. I feel they've had a better time at home.' Others spoke of their sense of strangeness upon return home: 'It felt a little as if the place was moved round or it wasn't the same house.' 'It seems different. The air you breathe is funny—so cool, and the breeze, you forget what a breeze felt like, being in the ward.'

Generally, such feelings of slight jealousy and difference seemed well contained and older children were not overly demanding upon their return home.

Relationship of fears, including hospital fears, to obvious illness symptoms

Generally, far from adapting to their ever-present and obvious illness symptoms—such as cough and wind—cystic children found them an increasing source of embarrassment and stress. This was especially true of older children who had to mix socially with their well peers. Physical attributes associated with the illness, such as being small and thin, or having teeth blackened by antibiotics, elicited taunts in school and produced understandable distress. For instance, a five-year-old said of his companions, 'They won't play with me. When I ask the children they turn their backs on me because I don't look nice.' A seven-year-old said, 'I'm just a stick-in-the-mud,' and a sixteen-year-old commented: 'I'm always thin. It annoys me when I get slagged about it. They call me Biafran. They just shout it at me and run.' In school, physical symptoms could cause distress in other ways; for example, a ten-year-old disliked 'having a cough because when you're writing it makes you scribble', and a seven-year-old said she hated 'coughing and sneezing. When the class is quiet I sneeze and everyone looks round.'

Even in the security of their own home, children displayed fears regarding their symptoms. Often they assessed their physical progress with reference to them, and when they realised they were not progressing satisfactorily this added to their overall distress. For example, a seven-year-old confided:

'I don't like coughing and seeing what I cough up. It's spittle. I hate spittle. It's phlegm. Mummy knows what I'm like by its colour. If it's white you're getting better. If it's grey you've got a cold. If it's yellow you're getting worse, and it worries me when it's yellow.'

Occasionally, unexplained symptoms fed frightening fantasies. For example, a five-year-old believed 'there's bugs inside me chest'. An eight-year-old said the worst things about being ill were 'being afraid, and thinking of things like there's an animal inside and it never goes away from me'. Such fantasies were especially frightening when the child felt guilt for causing his symptoms, either by going outside into the cold, or by refusing his treatment, or failing to eat. For example, a six-year-old told me he had a bad chest which worried him because he got it 'by going into the street, and staying out too late'. Parents often unwittingly contributed to this fantasy by describing the sick child as 'being taken bad' or having a 'bad' symptom, which the listening child then associated with being naughty.

Whilst less severe symptoms stimulated such fears, the more serious symptoms often produced near panic, both on the part of the parents and possibly because of this—on the part of the child. Twenty-two per cent of the fifty-eight children I observed suffered occasionally from bowel prolapse, the lower part of the bowel suddenly projecting from the child's body. Parents recollected their distress when this first occurred: 'He was sitting on his pot and he started to yell and scream and when my husband looked his back passage had collapsed. We were terrified and we took him up to hospital straight away.' The mother of a four-year-old girl said: 'She panicked a bit and I had to go in and get the lady next door. She is a panicky child and when she panics I panic all the more and get all worked up.' Another four-year-old 'was on the toilet and she screamed. I had no idea. Even our doctor didn't know what to do. Now she gets very hysterical about it, really upset about it.' The appearance of such a dramatic and unexplained symptom seemed to have a traumatic effect on the parents, and markedly changed their behaviour subsequently. Thus the parents of children with bowel prolapse reported more fears for their children's survival, and when they were hospitalised visited them significantly more often than parents of children without this symptom.*[1]

Similarly, children with this symptom were significantly more fearful in terms of their general behaviour at home compared with cystic children without bowel prolapse.[2] In terms of their protest behaviour and fearfulness in hospital, children who suffered from bowel prolapse were significantly more disturbed in the hospital environment than other cystic children.[3]

The association between the child's apparent fearfulness, his protest behaviour in hospital and his treatment protest behaviour at home

Whilst most children exhibited some emotional and behavioural discomfort in response to their illness, their home-based therapy and their hospital admissions, some children exhibited consistently more fearfulness in all spheres. Thus school-age children described by their parents in terms of their behaviour at home as being 'very fearful or 'moderately fearful' had higher scores on an objective measure of anxiety (the Taylor Manifest Anxiety Scale) than children described as 'showing very little fear'.[4]

Equally, children of all ages who were described as 'very fearful' or 'moderately fearful' were thought to show significantly more

* Differences between groups were assessed using the t test.
[1] $t = 2.04$, df $= 56$, $p < 0.05$.
[2] $t = 3.06$, df $= 55$, $p < 0.01$.
[3] $t = 2.09$, df $= 56$, $p < 0.05$.
[4] $t = 3.11$. df $= 7$, $p < 0.05$.

general response to their illness than children showing 'very little fear'.*[1]

In hospital, children who were 'very fearful' or 'moderately fearful' displayed significantly more protest behaviour than children showing 'very little fear'.[2]

Similarly, upon return home fearful children exhibited more behaviours indicative of distress than children who showed very little fear.

Conversely, those children who protested least in hospital protested least following it.[3]

These observed relationships force one to the conclusion that a small number of children are consistently fearful whenever stressed, whether the stresses are due to illness or hospital experiences.

Relationship between child protest behaviour in hospital and treatment protests at home

Just as some children would seem more consistently afraid than others whenever stressed, so also some children would appear to protest consistently against their environment whenever it was disliked. There was thus a tendency for children who protested most about their home-based treatment to protest most when hospitalised.[4]

To some extent, protests in both spheres might be related to sheer frustration produced by the restraints of treatment. In this respect, there emerged a fairly consistent relationship between the number of treatment procedures required by the child at home, and the number of protest behaviours he exhibited in hospital. Thus the child who had to bear most in terms of home-based therapy displayed most frustration and protest behaviour in hospital.[5]

---

* Differences between groups were assessed using the t test.

[1] $t = 2·69$, df $= 52$, $p < 0·01$.

[2] $t = 2·74$, df $= 44$, $p < 0·01$.

[3] $t = 3·09$, df $= 33$, $p < 0·01$.

[4] $t = 4·65$, df $= 4$, $p < 0·01$.

[5] $t = 2·78$, df $= 25$, $p < 0·02$.

8

Practical problems posed by chronic disease

'Sometimes I get wearied out looking after him, but I would want to be caring for him myself. It would be a lot harder for me if I wasn't caring for him. I would worry too. I just love him and like doing things for him.'

(*Mother*)

Having a chronically sick child in the family inevitably poses some practical problems for parents. Domestic chores are interrupted or postponed in order to provide time for treatment. Visits to out-patient clinics—though necessary—may interfere with parental work routines, and, on a long-term basis, prove costly and disruptive. Feeding and clothing a child with special needs can prove difficult for those on a limited budget. Housing problems may be highlighted by the need to provide space for bulky equipment. In addition, by putting further strain on the parents, such practical problems may accentuate physical and emotional upset consequent on diagnosis.

Despite the enormous importance of recognising and alleviating such problems, few attempts have been made to gauge their extent in the United Kingdom. Perhaps it is thought that practical difficulties consequent on chronic disease are largely diminished in a welfare state. This may be true, but, none the less, where they exist they can be very damaging to the general wellbeing of the families who sustain them. Certainly in North America and Australia great stress is laid on the detrimental effects of financial and housing difficulties arising from the illness of one family member (McCollum (forthcoming), Beveridge and Lykke, 1973). There, all family members are thought to suffer from the extensive drain on domestic resources which chronic illness represents.

As a first step to ascertaining the extent of some practical problems associated with the diagnosis of a chronic childhood disease, questions were included relating to housing, financial and work difficulties in the three questionnaires used with the parents of cf children.

Housing difficulties associated with cf

It is often argued that cf families encounter problems in housing the child's equipment, especially the mist tent (McCollum, forthcoming). Study parents were therefore asked a series of questions concerning the extent and nature of their domestic accommodation, their feelings of satisfaction or dissatisfaction concerning this, and, most especially, the need for modifications required to house adequately the sick child or his equipment.

Generally, in Northern Ireland, housing problems due solely to the child's illness were slight. Although 24 per cent of mothers reported that their present house did not fully meet their family's needs, upon closer inspection it was found that such housing inadequacies existed before the child's illness and were merely exaggerated by it. For example, 8 of the 53 families had no inside flush toilet, 6 had no bath, 4 had no hot water system and 1 no running water. Naturally, all these inadequacies hindered the mother's ability to cope satisfactorily with her family's washing, bathing, and toileting, and the need for better facilities became even more pressing after the birth of a child in need of very special care. None of these difficulties was created by the sick child, however, all were present before his birth and were merely accentuated by it.

Seventeen per cent of mothers felt that they needed more space with a sick child, but again those who experienced this feeling were those who were already severely pressed for space, and the advent of any new baby, whatever his physical condition, would have posed such a problem. However, housing a sick child may have made some mothers more aware of domestic deficiencies. Whereas with a well baby the mother might have persuaded herself that she could manage, a delicate child could not be expected to sustain the same spatial deprivations, and the birth of such a child made the home seem more inadequate.

Sixty per cent of cystic children in this study shared their bedroom. In 25 per cent of cases they shared with their parents. Occasionally, sharing was necessitated by lack of space; for example, one little girl had to share her bed with her well sister, whilst three other well siblings slept in another bed in the same room. Most usually, however, sharing was arranged to meet the emotional needs of the child or his parents, and would have taken place whatever the size of the domestic dwelling. For instance, one farming family, who lived in a rambling farm house, genuinely believed that the sick child was 'too delicate to be put out on his own', and at the time of the study—when he was ten—he was still sharing his parents' double bed.

Financial difficulties associated with cf

In the American and Australian literature, great emphasis has been placed on the drain imposed on a family's financial resources by the need to provide medication and medical care for a cystic child in a non-welfare state (McCollum, forthcoming; Teicher, 1969; Beveridge and Lykke, 1973). Instances have been cited in which both parents needed to take two jobs apiece in order to meet the excessive costs of inpatient treatment, routine X-rays, medicines and regular check-ups. As a consequence, the parents were deprived of leisure, and the whole family lost necessary opportunities for relaxation together.

Whilst, in a welfare state such as that in Northern Ireland, I did not expect to find such serious financial deprivations, I was nevertheless curious to know exactly how much the average cystic child cost his parents to maintain each year, and what were the actual financial strains imposed by the disease.

Several issues seemed worthy of consideration: first, the cost of transport to the out-patient clinic: second, the additional cost of feeding a frequently hungry child, who in some instances required a high-protein diet; third, the cost of extra clothes; fourth, the loss of earnings occasioned by absence from work when the child was sick; and, finally, additional expenses such as increased electricity charges due to running the mist tent.

Briefly, the survey showed that in Northern Ireland 73 per cent of families required regular transport to the out-patient clinic, the remaining families either walking or being taken there by ambulance. Transport costs ranged from 50p to £12 per annum—the average cost being £3.50.

Forty-five per cent of families felt obliged to buy extra milk or better foodstuffs for the sick child, and the cost of these foods ranged from £6 to £100 per annum, the mean being £57.

Only 13 per cent of families bought better clothes for the sick child. Mothers found it hard to estimate how much more they spent on these items but the average additional cost was thought to be around £20 per annum.

Whilst 22 per cent of families had their work patterns disrupted by cf at one time or another, only 11 per cent of workers had actually lost their earning power temporarily because of it. Losses occasioned by such workers ranged from one week's pay of £25 to three months' pay valued at £308. The average loss to families sustaining such deprivation was a total of £125, or approximately £25 per annum for each year of the sick child's life.

Finally, an assessment was made of additional expenses incurred in diverse ways; for example, the cost of visiting the sick child in hospital, and the cost of providing extra heat in his room during the winter months. Twenty-two per cent of families sustained such expenses, and these averaged £14 per annum.

When the total cost of illness expenses was calculated for each family, considerable individual differences in expenditure were apparent. At one extreme, nine families thought they spent nothing extra because of the illness, whilst on the other hand two families were thought to spend in excess of £150 per annum (Figure 2 gives details of the exact incidence of additional annual expenditure sustained by the study families).

On average, each study family spent an additional £39 per annum on each cf child (range = £0-£250). Overall, this would not seem an excessive burden. However, in those few instances where expenditure was markedly high some financial discomfort was certainly apparent. In addition, in cases where the father was unemployed or poorly paid, and financial stresses were severe, the parents' ability to cope adequately with the child and his illness seemed much diminished.

In one such family, the father was earning £18 a week net when I first spoke to him. On this he supported himself, his wife and his

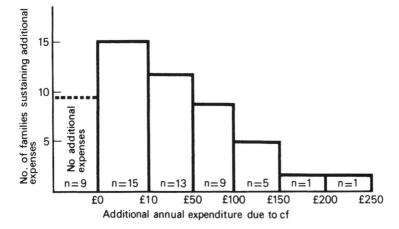

Figure 2   *Incidence of additional annual expenditure sustained by study families due to the illness*

four children. His wife was unable to work because the sick child genuinely needed constant day and night attention. The family rented a house which cost £2.50 a week. Because they lived in a rural area, fifteen miles from the father's work, they were obliged to run a car. This they bought on hire purchase, costing £2 a week. In addition, the mother incurred an extra hire purchase commitment in buying a washing machine needed to launder the vast quantity of bedding and clothing soiled daily by the incontinent child. Every month the father had to forgo half a day's work to take the child for his regular clinic check-up. When the child was hospitalised, which he was on average twice a year, the mother could not afford the return bus fare of 50p to go and see him every day. The family had never had even a day's outing, let alone a holiday. Meals were skimped, hurried affairs, lacking in protein, especially in meat. The mother regularly did without.

At the time of my initial interview, when the child was six, the family spent an additional, and ill-afforded, £81 per annum on the sick child. Family morale was in tatters, with the mother verging on a nervous breakdown and the father antagonistic to all medical and social work personnel. Not surprisingly, the child's symptoms, treatment and daily care had become foci for the expression of their general economic frustration. Both parents constantly scolded the child, who responded by becoming withdrawn, depressed and non-cooperative, most especially in terms of his treatment.

More recently, the introduction of the Family Income Supplement, the obtaining of an Attendance Allowance and the provision of a free annual holiday by the Cystic Fibrosis Research Trust have done much to combat these difficulties. Both parents appear less strained, they display only minimal resentment and are more ready to seek and accept medical advice. The child's health has improved, and he has remained outside a hospital ward for a longer period than at any other time in his existence.

Work problems for parents associated with cf

The mothers Caring for a chronically sick child in the home is a time-consuming and worrying affair. It seemed probable therefore that many study mothers would have experienced serious setbacks in their domestic work because of the illness, or felt themselves deprived of opportunities for assuming paid employment outside the home. These possibilities were therefore investigated.

Surprisingly, upon questioning, only a handful of mothers reported experiencing any lasting difficulties in accomplishing their domestic tasks. Their success in this respect seemed due to two factors. First, they generally made the sick child's care their first concern, and expected correspondingly less of themselves in terms of domestic efficiency. 'The child comes first. The house can go to pot as long as he is looked after.' 'If I get my housework done, I get it done. If I don't, I don't.' Second, with the exception of only six mothers who were either geographically isolated from their families or emotionally isolated from friends by denying husbands, every mother I questioned had some additional source of practical help available if she required it.

Most usually, additional domestic help came from the mother's immediate family—her own mother, her sisters, or, very occasionally, her in-laws. Seventy-one per cent of mothers questioned had such family members living within walking distance of them. Of the remainder, the majority had family living within travelling distance who could be relied upon to help if needed. From the spontaneous comments of most mothers, it was obvious that family members were a great source of strength and practical assistance offering whatever services were required. 'They're that good, they'd do anything. They'd do the housework or babysit.' 'My mother would always keep them, all night if we want to go out. My family would do anything, even the washing, if I'm stressed.' 'They're the only ones I would think of leaving the child with—they have him spoilt. They look after him really well.'

Even in cases where family members had never actually been asked to do anything, the knowledge that they were there, and could be absolutely relied upon if needed, was a great comfort for many parents.

Only 9 per cent of mothers were without such family support. In all instances they were émigrés to Northern Ireland, women whose husbands were working there only temporarily.

In addition to the practical help provided by relatives, 50 per cent of Ulster mothers accepted occasional help from friends or neighbours. In this respect also many mothers spoke very warmly of the assistance they were given and it was obviously of considerable emotional benefit to them to be accepted by, and receive such support from, the wider community. 'My next door neighbour is very good. She would babysit or shop, or if the child vomited she would change him from the skin out.' 'The woman next door would do anything for me. On this street you'd never be without help.' 'The neighbours are brave and good round here. I've known them since I was a youngster.'

In all, 89 per cent of Ulster mothers were given practical help of one sort or another by their family or friends. Usually this took the form of babysitting or caring for well children whilst the mother accompanied the sick child to the clinic, or visited him in hospital. In addition, about one-third of the mothers regularly relied upon relatives or friends to help with their domestic routine.

A third of the mothers said that at times, for example, when the child was unwell, they had to omit regular domestic chores such as ironing or cleaning. Usually they caught up with such tasks at weekends when their husbands were at home to look after the child. The most serious practical problem for mothers of cf children was the problem of shopping. Forty-five per cent of mothers were unwilling to take the child out in cold or wet weather, or into crowded places. Sometimes this problem was solved by the mother doing the bulk of the family shopping on Saturday when she could leave the child at home with her husband. She then relied on neighbours for the purchase of small items during the week.

Thirty-one per cent of study mothers worked outside the home, but only a quarter of these women said they had ever experienced difficulties in holding down a job whilst adequately caring for the sick child. As with their attitude to housework, mothers showed evidence of altering their expectations for themselves in the light of their commitment to the sick child. Whereas previously they might have expected more from themselves in terms of achievement, in view of the illness they were content with less, and, as with domestic chores, they put the child's welfare first. Family members were also of immense value, often acting as full-time housekeepers in the mother's absence.

For many mothers, work—whether domestic or outside the home—was of considerable therapeutic value. By cleaning out the home, or actively engaging in some outside pursuit, mothers were temporarily enabled to overcome their depression or forget some of their responsibilities. One country mother described it this way: 'When the child is really sick, I go down to the byre and cry. Then I do some work with the animals. It gives me an interest. I can't abide to be sitting. There'd be too much time for brooding.'

Thirteen of the thirty-six mothers who were housebound said they would like an outside job, but only two of them felt prevented from getting one because of the child's illness. The rest refrained simply because they felt their children were too young to permit them to leave home.

The fathers   In contrast to the wives, most of whom managed to work most successfully despite the illness, 40 per cent of the fathers interviewed felt that their work had been interfered with or negatively influenced by the child's illness. Generally, this interference was attributed to worry over the child's health, and seemed especially prevalent in men who worked on their own; for example, long-distance lorry drivers who had overmuch uninterrupted time to dwell on the problem. As one father commented: 'Every day at work I ponder over what is going to happen—studying this and that. You can't say you're a free man.' Worries of this sort were accentuated during times of crisis: 'When she went into hospital I felt like taking a week off. I just got a sickening feeling and found it very hard to settle to work.' The company of sympathetic work mates did much to alleviate such worries, but occasionally men had to be removed from hazardous work situations because their anxieties made it difficult for them to concentrate; for instance, one father said: 'I was depressed about the illness. The foreman took me off the machine at the time for my mind was wandering.'

Some fathers found that their worries increased during working hours because, away from home, they felt themselves deprived of the opportunity to care for the child. One typical father commented: 'I just love to be with him all the time, but I must go to work. There's nothing I can do about it.' In all, 26 per cent of fathers interviewed said that they wished they could be at home more often to help care for their child. This was especially true of fathers who worked some distance away from home.

Twenty-seven per cent of fathers had had to give up work at some time in order to care for the sick child or the family. Generally, such absences represented a financial loss and, in two cases, the father felt they prejudiced his career opportunities. Three fathers actually stayed in hospital with the sick child because their wives had to remain at home with other children. Whilst these fathers welcomed rather than resented this task, they none the less found that it created some work difficulties for them.

General hardships associated with cf

In North America it is generally believed that chronic illness is invariably accompanied by general hardship for parents. Because I felt that such hardships might more truly emanate from the economic privations produced by the illness rather than from the need to care for a sick child, I questioned the study parents carefully concerning their feelings of general deprivation.

Sixty-two per cent of mothers and 37 per cent of fathers admitted that the illness had produced some hardship for them. The disparity between the sexes in this respect undoubtedly mirrors the fact that in Northern Ireland mothers do shoulder the greater burden of caring for the sick child, and they are more deprived because of it.

Table 20 gives details of the incidence of some of the more common deprivations mentioned by parents. Lack of energy was a major problem for mothers, with almost half the group sustaining some loss. Generally, mothers acknowledged the existence of, but did not resent, this hardship; for instance, one mother commented: 'Sometimes I get wearied out looking after him, but I would want to be caring for him myself. It would be a lot harder for me if I wasn't

Table 20 *Parents experiencing hardships due to cf*

Hardship	Mothers (%)	Fathers (%)
Less energy	44	8
Less spare time	34	13
Less fun in life	32	17
Less spare time with spouse	24	17
Less money to spend on self	20	11
No.	52	45

caring for him. I would worry more. I just love him and like doing things for him.'

Similarly, about a third of the mothers, but only a small number of fathers, acknowledged that they had less spare time and less fun in life because of the illness. One mother described it this way: 'Whenever you go out he's always on your mind, and you wonder if you do go out will they cover him and keep him dry and make sure he comes to no harm.' In the same vein, a father remarked: 'Certainly we have less fun in life, because even if you're out you wonder how he's getting on, is he sick tonight or coughing.' However, most parents adapted to the illness and found that, despite it, they could still lead something approximating to a normal social life. Illustrating this, one mother confided: 'When we thought about him at first, we felt we could never be happy again. We wanted him so much—but it is amazing how you adapt to these things.'

Of least consequence was the loss of spending money due to the illness. Perhaps in Northern Ireland the overall cost of the illness was too slight to be much of a trouble to most families, or perhaps by contrast to other stresses and anxieties the loss of some personal pin money seemed the very smallest concern. Certainly, in this respect, Ulster parents are more fortunate than their equivalents in other communities. Beveridge and Lykke (1973) found that financial pressures occupied a 'leading position' in the sources of stress for cf families in Australia, and McCollum and Gibson (1971) emphasised the substantial financial deprivations encountered by similar families in the USA. The parents I spoke to were not oblivious of these facts, as one mother commented: 'I'm glad I'm living under a British flag and I have a health service. If I was in Eire or America, I wouldn't have that marvellous health service.' Such positive thoughts certainly assisted parents in coming to terms with the disease.

Ulster parents were also assisted in their adaptation to the illness by the fact that few of them had any startling ambitions, or even any clear picture of what they hoped to accomplish in their adult life. The majority seemed content, as one father expressed it, 'to go on as we're living now; paying our way and keeping out of trouble'. Such relatively unambitious aims made it possible for parents to accept the sick child and his illness without any great sense of socio-economic deprivation. Consequently, parents tended to minimise the practical discomforts and hardships which the situation produced.

9

Talking about the disease

'At times I'm sitting there and he says, "What are you worrying about?" and I say "Nothing," and he says "Yes you are," and I say "I'm thinking about John" and then he says nothing, for I think he knows he would worry me more if he agreed. . . . I can talk about most things with him, but not the illness. His mother thinks I should but I think what's the use of both of us worrying. He does care, he does understand, and that's enough.'

(Mother of a three-year-old)

Parenthood poses innumerable and often complex problems for the individuals concerned. At each stage in the child's development issues arise which necessitate decision-making. Parents must decide how best to train physical skills, how to develop social competence, how to potentiate emotional growth, and when and how to begin formal education. They must determine at what age to impart basic information relating to crucial life situations, and how best to answer the child's questions concerning himself, his abilities and his limitations. Such decisions challenge parents, most especially parents of children whose development is essentially non-normal. For them there is no easily available set of child-rearing rules to follow. Because their child is unique in terms of his symptoms, handicap or shifts in wellbeing, normal standards or orthodox training procedures may seem inappropriate. Informal advice, whether gleaned from family, friends, the mass media or child-care manuals, may similarly seem of little value; and expert help, whether that of the paediatrician, the GP, or the health visitor may not be immediately available. Consequently such parents must face many child-rearing issues alone, without additional sources of reference to guide their decisions.

As a result one might expect that parents of sick and handicapped children would display an elevated level of communication concerning the many child-orientated difficulties which face them. But this is not so. Quite the reverse. Such parents often exhibit a diminished level of communication, appearing to avoid, rather than foster, discussion. As early as 1964, Turk wrote of cf families being 'locked in a web of silence'. Five years later Kulczycki and his colleagues (1969) noted 'varying degrees of discomfort about talking' of cf in twenty families they studied. They also noted 'little or no discussion of feelings' amongst family members. Tropauer and his co-workers (1970) noted similar difficulties and Pinkerton (1969) concluded that such reticence might adversely affect older sick children, subjecting them 'to a comfortless state of utter loneliness, cut off from emotional communication, consumed by fear of the unknown, the victim of agonizing doubts'.

Whilst most of these observations were made in the USA, in a social climate markedly different from our own, it was interesting to find that many of the study families experienced exactly comparable communication difficulties. Sixteen per cent of women and 25 per cent of men said they were unable fully to talk over the illness with one another. Thirty per cent of women and 65 per cent of men said they were unable to discuss it fully with their kin, and with increasing social distance communication diminished still further (Table 21).

Generally men seemed less able than women to verbalise their feelings fully, and medical advisers were used as confidants by only a very small percentage of parents, women being more inclined to speak to them than men. This latter finding probably reflects the fact that in Northern Ireland mothers were most often present at therapeutic interviews, whilst fathers rarely attended.

Communication between spouses

Parents who were able to share their worries concerning the illness stressed two essential advantages of such communication. First, it

Table 21 *Parents who felt unable fully to communicate about cf*

	Women (%)	Men (%)
With spouse	16	25
With family	30	65
With friends	54	63
With GP	70	91
With paediatrician	68	93
No.	52	45

had a definite therapeutic value, lightening the emotional burden: 'It seems to get something off my chest.' 'It's good to talk, it helps me, rather than have it bundled up inside. It helps me for my own sake.' 'I don't hide anything for I feel if you're open it helps everyone to cope and understand. I feel if you keep it to yourself it tends to make you worry and be awkward and cross with the rest of the household.' 'It would go for your nerves if you didn't talk.'

In addition, full communication deepened marital relationships. One such couple admitted that in 'the first few days after he was diagnosed we talked of little else. We tried to sort out how much of our sadness was for us and how much for him. This helped us both greatly.' Communicative parents often gave each other courage, for example one father said: 'My wife has always been very strong. I think I'm a pessimist and she's an optimist. His life has never been in any doubt as far as she is concerned and it is always reassuring. She can rise above it easier than me, and I can lean on her in that respect. She's always been unchangeable in feeling he will surmount his difficulties.' Similarly, one partner often helped the other to come to terms with the illness by offering some acceptable explanation for the presence of cf in the family.

In contrast, the small minority of parents who were unable to talk over the event together frequently intimated that this silence had a limiting effect on their marriage, tending to divide, rather than draw them closer together. This was especially true where one partner was definitely desirous of communication but deprived of this by the denial processes of the other. For instance the wife of a man who 'likes to forget about the illness' said: 'I don't discuss it much. If you say much to my husband it annoys him. He won't tell his family and he won't let me tell them. I don't say much about it. I just get on with things on my own.' Another woman commented:

'My husband is afraid of me getting too much upset. He would say of those books [CF Trust leaflets] "For God's sake, won't you put them on the fire. You're better not seeing them." He wouldn't see them. He wouldn't read them himself. He says there's no point in reading something like that, it does no good. He won't give me the *C.F. News,* he burns it.'

Parents who admitted an inability to communicate concerning cf often justified this reticence in terms of their desire to spare the partner further worry: 'I keep on the bright side to keep her happy.' Occasionally they avoided the topic because it produced arguments: 'Sometimes she has a fatalistic view of the illness getting worse, and says the doctors are no good, and then I argue with her.' 'He listens sometimes but maybe wouldn't be very communicative about it and then he would shout "All right, all right, you don't have to go into it."' In addition, partners occasionally cited either their own inherent inability to communicate or their ignorance as an explanation for such silence: 'I don't talk much about it. I keep it to myself. I worry more inwardly than I would show. I do that with other things too. It's just my nature.' 'The two of us didn't know much about it. We haven't spoken of it much because we didn't worry about it.'

Communication between parents and other adults

As noted previously, full communication between parents and other adults decreased with social distance. Many reasons were advanced to explain this. First, parents expressed a desire not to worry family and friends unnecessarily. Often, as a result, parents evolved a policy of 'talking about his treatment but not about the fears we would have for his future'. Second, the desire not to be additionally worried by the negative reactions of others: 'I can only talk it over with my mother. My mother is very understanding but my mother-in-law makes it a thousand times worse. She worries me a lot more.' Third, the fact that so few people knew of the disease: 'No one really understands. No one knows anything about it.' 'My parents don't fully understand—whether or not they don't want to understand or are incapable of it I don't know. It's very difficult.' Fourth, many parents felt themselves in danger of boring others by constantly referring to their child: 'If people say, "How is the baby?" I don't go into details. I'm conscious of boring people so I don't discuss it at great length. But if there are follow-up questions I answer them.' 'It's nothing to be ashamed of, just an illness like everything else. Well, I used to be obsessed with cf. There was a point I was even telling the doctor the things he was leaving out. Sometimes, it's a good thing, sometimes not. Sometimes if you're less intelligent you get through better. I think too many things. My mind's too bright. You burden people. I don't mind talking to my husband and my family, but if you go on too much people get fed up and say, "I've got my own problems." People are involved in their own lives and you just have to cope with this illness in your own way.' Much the same reason was advanced by some parents to explain their inability to communicate fully with medical advisers: 'They're always very busy in the hospital. They never have time to talk. The assistants and the nurses give you more information than the doctors.'

Finally, some parents stressed the dangers inherent in communicating too fully with those whom they could not fully trust. One mother remarked: 'They might gossip.' Another explained: 'It does help me to confide in someone but you can say too much. My boy came in the other day and said, "That wee fellow down there said I'm going to die with my chest. He said I won't live past twenty." They'd seen an article saying these children would get worse when they get older and they'd die before twenty. It was not a nice thing to tell anyone.' Another mother confided:

'We don't discuss it very often now. My husband and I might discuss it together but not with others. You see we did take the child to a faith healer once and my husband told him it was a fatal illness and would kill the child, and the child heard and started to cry and wouldn't stop, and so since then we haven't discussed it with anyone.'

Parent-child communication

Any problems encountered by parents in talking to other adults about cf were slight compared with those they experienced in talking about the disease with their sick children. When the level of parent-child communication was assessed (allowing for age-appropriate differences in level of comprehension) only 27 per cent of the parents of school-age children were thought to communicate well with the sick child concerning his illness, a third had a moderate standard of communication, and 40 per cent of parents were poor communicators.

Generally, good communicators were drawn from the ranks of those who were able to assess realistically the effect of the illness on the child. They therefore faced up to the relevant issues and saw the need to arm the growing child against self-doubts and the insults of peers, by warning him in advance of his limitations. As one father observed: 'It's better to tell them. Like the orphan boy, tell them before they go to school or someone else will tell them.' Such parents frequently emphasised the need to keep illness communications natural, and to make them, wherever possible, a two-way affair, with the child freely asking questions, and offering comment:

> 'We've begun to talk sensibly with her. I think we've begun to get better understanding between each other. I feel we are no longer telling her, but talking around the subject. This encourages them to talk to you about what they feel.'

In contrast, various reasons were advanced to explain more limited communication, the most frequent being the parent's desire not to hurt the child. For example, one mother said: 'I'm a bit worried when it comes to talking to her about cf. I don't know whether I'll be able to and I don't want to harm her in any way. I feel I could harm her by saying the wrong things.' A father commented: 'It's a thing I'm dreading having to explain to him. It's not I don't want to explain—it's just what is the right way to put it over best.' Another mother attributed her reticence to advice from her family:

> 'There's my aunt who had two boys who died of multiple sclerosis and she says its better not to talk too much about it, because it upsets them. They walked until they were seven, and they died at sixteen and seventeen, and they never asked about why they didn't walk. They never asked questions. My aunt gives me good advice. She feels its better not to talk about it for it makes the children worry too. They sit and worry about it then.'

The incurable and potentially fatal nature of cf proved immense stumbling blocks to communication. Parents who might otherwise have been able to impart a few basic facts, found themselves terrified when they contemplated these threatening aspects of the disease, thus two fathers commented:

'It will be difficult—like breaking the news of a death sentence to someone. Telling her she's going to have it all her life, there's no hope of a cure. Telling her the length of it would disturb me.'

'We were told by the consultant that the child would not live beyond five and that this was the normal life expectancy nowadays. There is a problem now in relation to what we should tell her. You can't just rush in and say, "You're not going to live beyond this year" and yet she is entitled to know. What would you tell her? There's no sense in only giving her half the truth. If you're going to say anything you've got to say the lot, or she'll wonder what you're hiding, won't she?'

Often parents endeavoured to control their apprehensions by waiting for the child to initiate the discussion: 'I've made up my mind—when he does ask, I'll tell him.' 'I haven't told him nothing—I'm waiting for his questions.' 'We answer questions as they come up—we always try to be prepared for the next step, but we don't take any action in initiating it.' However, as many parents pointed out, in such circumstances the child frequently failed to ask questions, and the parent was forced either to sit him down and say 'Come on boy, I've something to tell you', or else to leave the subject for another year. Most opted for this latter course. As a result, few children were fully informed concerning their illness, for example when one considers the issues discussed by the mother with her cf child (Table 22) one finds that while two-thirds of the school-age children were able to talk over most non-illness topics naturally with their mother, and 76 per cent of such children asked questions about cf, only about half the children knew what the illness was called, and only about a third knew they would have it for life. Only one child out of the entire group had been told that the disease was inherited. Often parents justified this lack of information by saying that there was 'time enough when he's older'. Many felt that there was little point in explaining potentially distressing, and undoubtedly complex issues with a child who might not live long enough for such issues to assume relevance. Whilst one can respect such feelings in effect they

Table 22 *Issues discussed by mother with cf child*

	Pre-school children (%)	School-age children (%)	All children (%)
Most topics naturally	10	66	39
Cf inherited	0	3	1·5
Cf could get worse	3	23	14
Born with cf	3	41	22
Cf lifelong illness	3	37	21
Name of illness known	3	55	29
Child's queries illness	9	76	45
No.	28	30	58

tended to isolate the child, not only depriving him of knowledge, but making the whole subject taboo. As will be mentioned in Chapter 11 such a taboo did not remove children's fears, but merely prevented communication, reassurance, and resolution. Occasionally older children reared in non-communicating families, undoubtedly began to feel shame concerning the disease, so that when eventually the parent felt obliged to talk of the illness, the child refused to listen. The mother of a fifteen-year-old, who had remained silent until the boy was in his teens, said: 'He doesn't do his treatment now for he doesn't want anyone to know. If you mention the illness at all, he's disgusted and shakes his head. Closes his eyes and shakes his head.' Sadly, in homes such as these, valuable opportunities were lost for reassuring the child at an earlier, more appropriate age, when his fears were not so great, and parental reassurance was more acceptable to him.

Factors militating against good parent-child communication

Several factors appeared to affect adversely the parents' ability to speak of the disease.

(1) Mothers who felt guilty about their part in causing the disease, communicated less well with their children than mothers who did not feel guilty.*[1]

(2) Fathers who felt their marriage was not strengthened as a result of their experiences with the disease, communicated less well with their children than fathers who felt their marriage was strengthened.[2]

(3) Parents who had lost previous children were less able to talk over the illness than parents with no previous child loss (see below, p. 218).[3]

In all these respects it was obvious that where a parent was emotionally discomforted by the illness to a marked degree his ability to communicate with his child concerning it diminished significantly.

Factors affecting the child's ability to speak of his illness

Just as the parents' ability to speak of the illness was significantly affected by feelings of psychological discomfort, so also the children's ability to communicate appeared to be affected both by the general level of communication in the home, and also by the degree of emotional discomfort they were sustaining. Several relationships were apparent.

(1) The actual extent of parental communication affected that of the child. Thus parents who were moderate communicators had children who communicated better than parents who were poor communicators.[4]

(2) The extent of parental communication affected the degree of knowledge concerning the illness displayed by the child. Thus parents who were good communicators had children whose knowledge of the illness was significantly better than that of children of poor communicating parents.[5] Similarly, parents who were

* Differences between groups were assessed using the t test.
[1] $t = 2.12$, df $= 44$, $p < 0.05$.
[2] $t = 3.45$, df $= 40$, $p < 0.001$.
[3] $t = 2.63$, df $= 36$, $p < 0.02$.
[4] $t = 5.25$, df $= 39$, $p < 0.01$.
[5] $t = 3.84$, df $= 33$, $p < 0.001$.

moderate communicators had children whose knowledge of the illness was significantly better than that of children of poor communicating parents.*[1]

(3) The child's level of communication concerning his illness was significantly related to his parents' level of understanding concerning the illness. Children who were good communicators had parents who understood the illness better than the parents of children who were moderate communicators.[2] Also, children who were good communicators had parents who understood the illness better than the parents of children who were poor communicators.[3]

(4) The child's level of communication concerning his illness was significantly related to the extent of his parents' change in attitudes and expectations for him. Children who communicated least well had parents who had changed most in their attitudes and expectations. Thus children who were unable to communicate freely concerning the illness had parents who showed a significantly bigger change in expectations than the parents of children who were either moderate[4] or good communicators.[5] Similarly children who were moderate communicators had parents who changed less in their attitudes and expectations than parents of children who were poor communicators.[6]

(5) Finally, the experience of previous child loss in the family and the parents' reaction to this affected the level of communication displayed by the sick child. Children from families with no previous child loss communicated significantly better than children from families with prior loss. [7]

One is forced to conclude that a few parents found extreme difficulty in talking about the illness. Generally such reticence emerged from, or co-existed with other indices of psychological discomfort such as a wish to deny the illness, a feeling of guilt concerning its causation, or a sense of profound marital tension. Generally such feelings precluded a complete understanding of the

---

* Differences between groups were assessed using the t test.
[1] $t = 2.41$, df $= 39$, $p < 0.05$.
[2] $t = 2.33$, df $= 27$, $p < 0.05$.
[3] $t = 3.66$, df $= 27$, $p < 0.01$.
[4] $t = 3.60$, df $= 16$, $p < 0.01$.
[5] $t = 2.49$, df $= 15$, $p < 0.05$.
[6] $t = 2.75$, df $= 25$, $p < 0.02$.
[7] $t = 2.21$, df $= 44$, $p < 0.05$.

illness, and such parents were correspondingly disadvantaged in terms of informing the child adequately concerning his condition.

Parents advanced many reasons to explain their hesitation in informing the child adequately, the most cogent being their fear of hurting him unnecessarily. Whilst it would be quite wrong to advocate a policy of 'telling all' in every instance, complete silence or embarrassed hesitation would seem to handicap the child additionally in terms of his understanding of the illness, his ability to speak of it, and most especially his ability to gain reassurance and emotional comfort.

10

Changing hopes and expectations for the sick child

'This illness is a very serious thing—but I don't think it should alter your way of dealing with a child—though subconsciously it does.'

(Mother of a six-year-old)

When parents begin to appreciate the significance of their child's symptoms, their relationship with him changes in many subtle ways. Initially they handle him with greater care, extend him greater patience, and worry more about the falls and bruises he sustains at play. Later, as the limiting nature of the illness becomes more obvious, parents are forced to adapt their hopes and expectations for him to accord with this new and disappointing reality. Inevitably, such adaptation involves relinquishing some of the fantasies and goals which unconsciously they have attached to him. As Tisza (1960) commented, whereas before diagnosis the child was 'the embodiment of a promise', upon learning of the illness, that promise is 'either gone or at least reduced in value'. Adapting to this fact is a painful process, generating additional frustration and depression.

Problems also arise for parents in formulating new hopes and expectations for the sick child. In doing this, they are forced to take account of the child's actual physical limitations and, in addition, they must assess his real potential for growth. While suitable allowances must be made for his handicap, parents must none the less stimulate the child to maximum achievement at a realistic level.

For most parents, it is a difficult task to strike this ideal balance between protecting the child and helping him to grow. Yet, unless such a balance is attained the whole child suffers. As with well children, what the handicapped child must learn is 'how to capitalize on his capabilities, and, at the same time, to accept his limitations' (Hewitt and Newson, 1970). His attainment in this can be helped or hindered by the attitude of his parents.

Parents differ markedly in their ability to effect a balance between growth and protection. Some display an exaggerated need to stress the child's 'normality' and to deny the presence of any limiting physical defects. Others ignore the child's actual potential for growth and see only doom and disappointment as his inevitable lot. Between these two extremes there are all varieties of adaptation.

The age of the child, his actual physical condition, and his own response to the illness influence the nature of the balance which his parents attain. Similarly, the underlying personality structure of the parents, the support they are able to offer each other, and their previous illness experiences contribute to the degree to which they stress growth as opposed to protection. Previous loss of a child assumes especial significance in this context, bereaved parents being significantly more often inclined to protect rather than encourage to growth.

In all these respects, parents of children with cf do not differ from parents of other handicapped or chronically sick children. They are forced to adapt their hopes for the child in view of his illness, and many also change in their expectations for, and behaviour towards, him.

Changing child-rearing methods because of the illness

Fifty-three per cent of the parents interviewed admitted that their handling of the sick child was affected by their knowledge of his illness. As a consequence, they treated him differently from their other children. A further 18 per cent denied that the illness made any difference, but upon subsequent questioning were actually found to behave differently to the sick child. In only 29 per cent of cases was the sick child treated as normal by both his parents.

When parents were asked about their ideal in terms of rearing the sick child, however, the majority stressed the need for normality, and believed that any marked change in attitude would probably be detrimental to the child's overall growth. In only a few extreme cases was the need for protection given greater accord than the need for growth. The findings of this study concur in this respect with those of Hewitt (1970) and Barsch (1968), who found, when considering the rearing of physically handicapped children, that most parents

'set about the business . . . according to whatever set of beliefs they held about child rearing in general, and few of them changed their basic set of beliefs, even in the face of difficulties encountered in their day to day practices.'

As a consequence, in many homes there was a considerable disparity between what the parents hoped to achieve in terms of child rearing and what actually occurred. Because of this, 44 per cent of parents admitted that they were not happy in their handling of the sick child, and this added to their overall sense of stress (a factor to be considered in greater detail later in this chapter).

Parents who seemed most secure and happy in their rearing of the sick child were those few who claimed that their child was definitely different, and argued that it was therefore ridiculous to treat him as normal. One such mother of a sixteen-year-old said: 'I mean to say, a normal child gets on, but with him the abnormality is there and it has to have attention—it must do.' Similarly, the mother of a five-year-old commented:

'People tell me he could lead a normal life but I don't believe it. I don't think the kind of childhood he is leading is normal. There are so many medicines and treatments in it; for example, he has to wake at seven now to have his physiotherapy and breakfast before he catches his special school bus at eight.'

These mothers believed that the right attitude to the illness was 'just to accept it. There's nothing you can do about it. You can't cure it. You can't change it. You just have to do the best you can for them.'

Parents who emphasised their sick child's 'difference' experienced few problems in matching their behaviour to their beliefs: 'You'd spend more time playing with them, talking to them and comforting them.' 'I do do things for her that I wouldn't do for the rest, and she plays on that.' Generally, such parents justified their protective behaviour in terms of the child's possible death or his weakness; for example, the mother of a six-year-old said: 'I have fought for her life and she has fought for it, and it's always at the back of my mind. I wouldn't want to lose her. You do have pity—no, it's not pity—it's a mother's love for a child who's not as strong as the rest.' A father added: 'He may not be here that long. You never know how long you'll have these children for. While they are here you have to make the most of them.'

Usually, a parent was quite happy about his handling of the child if his behaviour and beliefs accorded in this way. Difficulties arose, however, if the marital partner was not in agreement with this over-protective attitude; for example, one mother confided: 'I feel, "God help her," but my husband says, "It's a hard world and she won't always have you."' Another mother, who had lost two previous children, said: 'My husband rears up about my spoiling the child. Perhaps it's a selfish attitude and not the right one to take, but I'll never have to look back and regret that I didn't have enough of him.'

At the other extreme, a few parents made no allowances for their child's handicap. Either they found themselves unable to accept that he was different, or they felt that any form of over-protection would be damaging to his growth. Thus the father of a six-year-old stated, 'I don't like making any differences for I think if I did she might think she was different from the rest, for I think if you pamper them they are inclined to put it on and make it worse for you and not good for themselves.' Occasionally, such parents had actually altered their rearing behaviour because they noticed that the sick child was beginning to take advantage of their leniency. The mother of an eight-year-old commented: 'Pampering doesn't help them. They need a fighting spirit if they're to do. I used to pamper her, and then I realised I made her sorry for herself, so I make her do things now.' Such parents denied treating their children in any way differently from normal, instead all their children were 'treated as equals'. They believed it right to treat a sick child 'just like any other, bring him up as a normal child, don't make any allowances for him, just let him go ahead'.

Often such parents demonstrated a determined optimism as far as the sick child's future was concerned, deliberately reminding themselves that the child could have an adult life: 'When she goes out into the world, she'll have to be treated the same as the rest. She's got all her faculties, she's not slow, so we treat her the same as the rest.'

'We try not to pamper her, we try to make her independent, so that if she gets up a bit and gets married, she can cope to a certain extent, and, in case anything happens to us, she can be independent and cope for herself.'

Occasionally, even such determined parents experienced difficulties in handling their children. Sometimes difficulties arose from character deficiencies on their own part and applied equally to all their children; for example, the mother of two boys, one well and one cf, said: 'I think I give in to them a bit too easily. I'm all for a quiet life. I hate crying and girning from both of them and would give in for quiet and my own enjoyment.'

Between the extreme attitudes of over-protection and inflexible equality lay a whole range of behaviours, which had normality as their ideal but none the less acknowledged the sick child's more vulnerable state.

Some parents gave their child his treatment, took extra care of his physical health and maintained a careful watch over him, yet in all other ways expected him to attain normal standards. Thus: 'with the exception of his treatment, which he has got to get, I make no difference between them. Everything else is on as equal a basis as possible, taking into account what he has.' The mother of a six-year-old, who encouraged most normal activities, said:

'If a cold or anything crops up, I'd be more worried and take more precautions, take more preventive measures, and I wouldn't take him into places where he could get cold, even a surgery where he might get germs, but I would like him to lead as normal a life as possible and I let him join activities or organisations away from home, though I might take a few precautions like putting on extra clothes and wellingtons.'

In other families, whilst the child was well he was treated normally, but parents altered their behaviour if he became ill; for example, the mother of a ten-year-old said: 'On the whole I treat him like the others, but when he's sick or depressed I give him more. I talk to him more.'

A few parents expected their child to behave normally within the home, but limited his freedom to go outside, fearing the effect of rain and cold on his health. For example, the father of a six-year-old said: 'We do definitely handle her differently. The wee boy gets out but she doesn't, or you take him a message, but not her, if the day is too bad. But you don't let them off with different things.' These parents stressed their fear of over-protecting the child. For them, protection was only justified in areas essential for the child's survival. Their ideal was to 'be aware of the threats—the things the child can't do because of his health—but on the whole to have as normal a parent-child reaction as you would with any other child'.

Inevitably, in some families natural concern for the child's physical wellbeing extended to include extra attention within the home, and, therefore, despite the parents' best intentions, there was a resultant difference in the quality of the sick child's life. Thus one mother commented: 'I try and treat him as normally as possible, but naturally they need that extra bit of attention from a normal child—but you try not to let him think he's different.' Obviously, there was a disparity between the way in which these parents would like to have reared their sick child and the way in which they were actually rearing him. Many parents admitted this openly: 'This illness is a very serious thing—but I don't think it should alter your way of dealing with the child, though subconsciously it does.' A few parents attempted to reconcile any observable disparity between ideal and reality by citing some additional characteristics of the child, which made protection imperative. One mother said: 'Unwittingly I do treat her differently. I don't mean to do it. I cuddle her more than the others, but she's a girl, and the youngest, and it is more appropriate.' The mother of a four-year-old explained:

'I have to treat her differently. She'd be more demanding than an ordinary child. If she wanted something you'd be more inclined to give it to her—more inclined not to refuse her. Whatever she wants, there and then, it has to be done—there and then, on the minute—or she lets go. She has a bad temper and if she has anything in her hand she would hit the other children.'

Parental unhappiness in child-rearing

Whilst acquiescing to demands of this sort many parents were distressed by their lack of firmness. In all, 44 per cent of parents said they were unhappy with their handling of the sick child; for example, one mother confided: 'You make an allowance—but I know I'm storing up problems for myself later, for there'll be a battle later.' The mother of a seven-year-old added: 'I feel I get trapped into doing things; for example, if he asked for sweets I'd give him them, rather than depriving him. There are quite a few things I'd give in to—maybe for peace—he's a great wee boy for getting his own way.' A father commented: 'I find sometimes that I should do things that I don't—for example, be his boss rather than let him boss me.' Similarly, the mother of an eight-year-old said: 'Often I find myself doing things that I don't approve of. I'm not happy at all with my handling of her, anything but. I'm treating her in ways I know are wrong—but to do it right seems impossible.'

For some parents, additional unhappiness and guilt resulted from their own impatience when provoked. The mother of a seven-year-old told me: 'One night he had a sore stomach and I'd been up with the other children and I went and shouted at him to go to sleep and then I lay awake about it and couldn't sleep.' Another mother commented: 'Sometimes I shout at her. There are times when she asks such silly questions and I've no patience. She asks the same questions a dozen times and I lose patience with her.' Several factors seemed to contribute to this irritability. First, parental ill-health following diagnosis: 'I don't reason as much as I should do. I'm always in a nervous state myself, tiredness mostly.' Second, worry concerning the child exaggerated natural concern: 'Sometimes I'm worried about her, and it plays on your nerves and it makes you feel responsible for her as if you should have kept her well. It plays on your nerves and you hit harder.'

Feelings of guilt on the part of parents following punishment of the sick child

Many parents experienced guilt and unhappiness after punishing the sick child for his naughtiness. This was especially true of parents of younger children. Sixty-seven per cent of parents of pre-school children and 50 per cent of parents of school-age children admitted to such feelings. As a result, punishment of the sick child placed many parents in a dilemma. It was obviously essential on a short-term basis to check the child lest he became out of control: 'I don't like being strict with her, but I find if I'm not there are problems. It's for her own good. I have to do things that I believe in rather than what I would like.' At the same time, faced with a potentially fatal disease, long-term objectives such as character formation seemed irrelevant, and many parents felt it unfair to burden the child additionally. For example, one father said: 'If he's done something he had to get smacked for he gets smacked, but afterwards when you think of his physical condition you have your doubts.' A mother commented: 'I feel if anything happened to him, if he should die—I don't think it's right he should get beat.'

Limiting punishment meted out to the sick child

Possibly because of their feelings of discomfort, 46 per cent of parents admitted that they were less likely to punish the sick child, even when justly provoked. In addition, some parents cited the adverse physical effect which punishment had on the sick child as a further reason for refraining from punishing him; for example, a father said: 'It brings on the coughing. You punish her, tap her on the hand, and she starts to cough, and it's too big a punishment.' He added: 'Her mother would chastise her now, and I would speak crossly, but we don't really hit her.'

In a few families the child had obviously seized upon this advantage, and, with impunity, had become increasingly naughty; for instance, the mother of a six-year-old said: 'If I went to hit her she would say, "Now you know I'm not well." '

Changes in the parents' expectations for the child

Besides changing rearing habits because of the illness, two-thirds of the parents admitted to altering hopes and expectations for the child. Most frequent were changes in hopes for the child's school achievement. About one-third of the parents expected less of the child in terms of basic school work because of his illness. This trend was especially apparent among the parents of older children, and obviously reflected their increasing awareness and sympathy for the child's physical limitations; for instance, the mother of a seven-year-old said: 'I feel she has enough with the illness to contend with, without pushing her.' The mother of a six-year-old who expected 'moderately less' of her in terms of school achievement said: 'If she wasn't doing well at school I wouldn't shout at her. I wouldn't expect a lot of her. I wouldn't keep on and on. She has enough worry of her own without putting worry into her.'

As with the parent's attitude to child-rearing generally, there was a considerable range in attitude towards school achievement. At one end of the continuum, a few over-protective parents had abandoned all scholastic aspirations; for instance, one mother who expected 'much less' of her daughter in school attainment said: 'I wouldn't care—we always say she needn't work at all. She can stay home and not work. I wouldn't push her at all. I'm not worried about school work as long as she progresses all right.' Similarly, the mother of a newly-diagnosed pre-school child commented:

'I wouldn't push him to learn. I wouldn't force him out to school. If he is unwell I'd let him stay at home and take the day off. I would never push him with his schoolwork for I feel if he is spared he can always stay at home with us.'

At the other end of the continuum, a few parents stressed the need to develop the child's intellectual abilities to 'compensate mentally for what he hasn't got physically'. Three sets of parents said they would actually push the child towards scholastic attainment. As one father explained: 'She will need her education more than most so we would encourage her to go as far on in school as she can.' A mother added: 'We would like him to get on well for it would help him to get an indoor job—an easy job.'

Between these two extremes there was a whole range of attitudes which emphasised growth as the ideal, but tempered hope with reference to reality: 'I expect a lot of her on the basis of her ability, but would be satisfied with less if she's not well.' Occasionally, parents admitted that the child played upon their concern—diminishing his own efforts accordingly: 'He's a bit fly at school. He puts the cough on and the teacher lets him off.' Undoubtedly, such subtle changes in the child's motivation affected performance in schoolwork, and it was not therefore surprising to find that all but one of the school-age study children were retarded in one or more basic school subject (the only exception being a child whose parents knew virtually nothing of the illness and, excluding his medicine, treated him as absolutely normal).

Twenty-four per cent of parents felt that their sick child would be less able to join in activities away from home. They advanced two reasons to support this change in their expectations. First, as one mother commented: 'I would be frightened of letting him go too far in case people didn't know how to handle him'; and, second, parents felt that activities away from home might involve the child in outdoor pursuits which could hazard his health. None the less, most parents agreed with the father who said: 'We would worry about him whilst he was away, but if he felt he was able we would let him go.'

Twenty-two per cent of parents were apprehensive about allowing the sick child to join normally in physical activities. They felt that such activities might hazard the child's health; for example, one mother said that sports might bring on her son's coughing. A father added: 'I don't think I would let her play hockey for it would be too much for her.'

Table 23   *Parents who changed in their expectations for the sick child*

Less expected of the sick child in terms of	Parents of children under five years (%)	Parents of children over five years (%)	Total group (%)
Keeping himself clean, neat and tidy	25	13	18
Helping with household chores	25	23	24
Success in schoolwork	25	36	31
Getting on well with other children	28	10	18
Being able to make his own independent decisions	18	16	17
Being able to join activities on his own, away from home	25	23	24
Being free to join in physical activities	25	19	22
No.	52	45	97

A few parents cited supposed conversations with the doctor in support of their attitude; for instance, the mother of a seven-year-old said: 'I keep her in as long as possible for the doctor said every cold would damage her lungs and she would have less of a chance and I'm inclined to keep her in to avoid damage.' When parents felt the doctor was in favour of protection they were more likely to protect. Conversely, where he emphasised the need for growth and experimentation they gained courage. Thus, the father of a three-year-old said: 'Our doctor said we should let him do what he's able to do. Physical activities would do him all the good in the world, especially for his lungs, football and trampolining.' Many parents stressed the need for the child to discover his own limitations for himself; for instance: 'He'll have to set the limits on his own. We'll let him set his own limits. He'll have to see what he can do on his own. If he wants to wrestle, we'll let him go right ahead and do it.'

Much the same attitudes prevailed in terms of allowing the child to make his own decisions. Most parents viewed independent decision-making as a necessary part of life, and only 17 per cent of parents felt constrained to override the child's own decisions because of their concern for his health. These parents stressed their need to prevent the child from undertaking tasks or activities which might prove too onerous for him; for instance, the mother of a seven-year-old said: 'She wanted to join the Brownies but I wouldn't let her join them for you have to go out at night, but I think if she gets this winter over, she'll be stronger and can go.'

Parents varied considerably in the degree to which they expected their sick child to help with household chores. Seventy-six per cent of parents expected him to help normally around the home. This, they felt, was only fair: 'If he's able to play, he's able to put away.' Some favoured domestic activities because they stimulated a necessary sense of independence in the child; for example, one mother said: 'I even make her do more things than my wee boy. I think they should be independent and able to do things for themselves. If you're going to do things for her it makes her special and puts her out of control.' Many parents were pleasantly surprised by the helpfulness of their cf children in the home; for instance, an eight-year-old was 'very domesticated. She goes out and washes her own socks.' Her mother added: 'I don't tell her to do it, she does it. She even goes and makes the beds.' The mother of a two-year-old, who actively encouraged the child to be independent, said: 'She's a busy bee, and wants to do things for herself.'

In this respect, as in others, much depended on parental attitude. The 24 per cent of parents who expected the child to do less in the home—'I wouldn't expect her to do anything at all'—were rarely disappointed; and several young children, subjected to such over-protection, had become tyrannical to the point of being unpleasant. As one mother said: 'She knows I will eventually do things for her. She shouts but she knows I will do it. She won't look for things herself, she says "Mummy, go and get it." Oh, I know it's my fault, it's the way I started her off.'

Parents were asked whether they expected less of their sick child in terms of keeping himself clean, neat and tidy. While a quarter of the parents of younger children expected less, only 13 per cent of parents of older children had changed their expectations in this respect. By contrast, most stressed the fact that the sick child was markedly neater and tidier than their other well children; for instance, a seven-year-old was 'a bit fussy about what clothes she puts on. Everything has to be very clean and so so. She's very fussy. She always washes her hands after the toilet. She's exceptionally clean. She can't stand other children with dirty noses and faces. She's always changing her pants.' Similarly, a six-year-old boy was described as 'very fussy, keeping himself always neat and clean. After lunch he washes himself and pulls his trousers up. He never leaves his trousers hanging down.' A seven-year-old boy had 'very expensive tastes—even in clothes. It was always the same. He's always been expensive and fussy. Now he wants suede boots with zips up them and a watch with the date on it.'

Whilst some parents welcomed and encouraged this fastidiousness, in other homes the sick child's longing for mod gear caused financial embarrassment and became a point of contention rather than rejoicing; for instance, the mother of a six-year-old girl who refused to wear 'ordinary clothes' said: 'She has this awful obsession about clothes. You feel you'd like to kill her at times. She dresses up. She wants to be in mod clothes, she wants to be a big girl in big girl's clothes.' Similarly, the father of a nine-year-old felt it a sad rather than joyful reflection on his son's overall development that he remained neater and cleaner than the rest of the brood: 'He's far neater and tidier than the others. He never dirties his clothes. If he did he would be a far better man. The rest were always out mucking and dirtying their hands. He's not that sort and never was.'

Perhaps by paying extra attention to their physical appearance, some sick children felt more socially acceptable. Personal fastidiousness could therefore be a defensive reaction, helping them to combat feelings of inadequacy engendered by the illness. In much the same way, some sick children took extra care to be helpful round the home, thus potentiating good relations between themselves and their parents.

Finally, parents were asked whether they expected less of their sick child in terms of his ability to get on with other children. Twenty-eight per cent of parents of pre-school children made extra allowances for the child in this way. By contrast, only 10 per cent of parents of older children admitted to such changes in expectation. A few parents attributed these changes to the uncompromising attitude of their sick child; for instance, a seven-year-old was 'selfish. He's not as generous as other children.' His father thought this due to the 'fact' that 'he always gets his own way in hospital'. A mother commented: 'I try and get her to be reasonable, but it's very difficult to manage. She's always very difficult.' She added: 'I only wish I could prevent her from fighting with the other two. She does play them up a lot.'

Where the sick child was allowed to dominate the home, tensions between brothers and sisters inevitably developed; for instance, the mother of a ten-year-old girl said:

'I expect them to give in more—especially the older girl has had to give in more. I know it's not fair to the others and yet you have to make allowances. I talked to my son about it, he's thirteen and he really resents it. I took him in and talked to him. I told him what she had. It was all right for a while, but now he doesn't seem to particularly like her—that sounds so awful—it did upset him when I told him, but he doesn't like her.'

Tensions between brothers and sisters added to the parents' difficulty in handling the sick child, engendering in them either a compensatory need to protect the sick child, or a sense of sadness for well children, and resentment at the sick child's demanding behaviour.

Agreement between spouses in changing expectations for the sick child

Each parent was asked individually whether he felt himself in agreement with his spouse concerning rearing methods and expectations for the sick child. Seventy-three per cent of parents agreed with each other about most things, though some added that one spouse was slightly stricter than the other. This finding concurs with that of Hewitt and Newson (1970) who found that 67 per cent of parents of cerebral palsied children were in close agreement with each other concerning child-rearing methods. They concluded: 'although it was evident that there was considerable disharmony in a few families, there was nothing to suggest that having a handicapped child made this more likely.' This conclusion is certainly true of the cf parents studied here. When the change in expectation scores[1] obtained for each spouse was compared with that of the married partner, only 34 per cent of couples differed substantially from one another. The most disparate couples had all lost previous children and it seemed that in such families one partner was still mourning for the dead child, and, consequently, over-protecting the remaining cf child, whilst the other partner had emerged from his grief and was more prepared to encourage the remaining sick child to growth and development. (Some argue that such dissonance in grieving is fairly widespread. Indeed it may be essential for the survival of the family, for if both parents were to mourn extensively there would be no one to care for the surviving children.)

Couples who differed fundamentally in their handling of and expectations for the child were additionally strained by this dissonance. For example, the mother of a three-year-old said: 'My husband is not strict at all, and it makes me mad at times. He says, "You're lucky to have the child, to have him here." Well, that's all right, but you can't let him off with everything.' The mother of a ten-year-old girl experienced the same difficulties:

'If I'm cross and send her upstairs, he would say, "Ah, she's not too well." It's difficult. I can see his point, and yet there are times she does things and you can't let it pass for the child's own sake. She's not always going to have people saying, "Ah dear, she's not too well, she can get off with this and that".'

---

[1] The change in expectation score was derived from the parents' responses to eight questions concerning changes in child-rearing habits or expectations for the child contained in the questionnaire. If parents agreed that they had changed in their expectations or behaviour towards the child, they were then asked whether they expected 'much less', 'moderately less', or 'only a little less of him' in terms of his accomplishments in this sphere. A score of 3 was allotted to the response 'much less', 2 to 'moderately less', and 1 to 'very little less'. Scores for individual items were then summated, the maximum expectation change score for each parent being 24. In forty-four families, both parents were evaluated in this way, and a gross parental change in expectation score was derived, the maximum score possible being 48.

Occasionally, parental quarrelling was noticed and played upon by the sick child. This then led on to even greater difficulties; for instance, one six-year-old had sleeping problems and while her mother tended to let her come down and spend the evening by the fire, her father insisted that she go back to bed, with the result that 'if we quarrel she takes my part, and then she won't let my husband forget it. This can go on for three weeks, with her looking daggers at her father. I say, "Forget it, it's all right," but it goes on.'

Change in expectations for the sick child according to the sex and social class of the parent

Where change in expectation scores were compared, mothers were found to change more than fathers in their expectations for the sick child. On average, the fifty-two mothers obtained an expectation change score of 4·5, whilst the forty-five fathers obtained a score of 3·2.

Similarly, when one compares the expectation change scores obtained by parents from different socio-economic groups (Table 24), one finds that mothers in the higher socio-economic classes appear to change their attitudes and expectations for the child more markedly than mothers in classes IV and V. This trend is also apparent—although less obviously—amongst the fathers.

To some extent, this greater change in expectation amongst better educated parents may reflect a greater general concern for the sick child on their part. Such concern also manifests itself in their greater speed in effecting diagnosis, the greater enthusiasm amongst such fathers to attend the diagnostic interview, their better knowledge of the illness, and their greater willingness to administer treatment to their child.

The association of previous child loss with the parents' change in expectation scores

As mentioned previously, parents who had already lost a child—whether from cf or from some other disease—changed most markedly in their expectations for the sick child. Table 25 gives the combined parental change in expectation score for forty-four sets of parents, both of whom were available for interview. From this one can see that twenty-six sets of parents with no loss had between them an average expectation change score of 8·0, being only half that for the seven sets of parents who had lost one child, and only about a quarter of that obtained by the parents who had lost three previous children. When these results were subjected to statistical analysis, a significant difference was found between the expectation change scores of couples who had sustained one loss, and those who were not bereaved of a child.[1]

Table 24 *Average change in expectation score according to the sex and social class of the parents*

		I and II	III M and III NM	IV and V
Mothers	Score	6·3	4·8	2·3
	No.	14	25	11
Fathers	Score	3·2	3·7	2·3
	No.	11	24	8

Many bereaved parents believed that protection was the only feasible attitude for them to take to another sick child; for example, a mother who had lost two previous children said her ideal was

'to treat them as well as ever you can, and give them everything you can that they want, and if they're sick spend all your time nursing them, talking to them a lot, trying to explain to them and making them understand, and trying to attract their mind away.'

Often such an attitude was exaggerated by feelings of guilt associated with supposed inadequacies in the parents' handling of the dead child. One mother who had lost two children expressed it this way:

Table 25 *Average parental change in expectation scores, according to the parents' previous experience of bereavement*

	No loss	One previous loss	Two previous losses	Three previous losses
Score	8·0	15·7	13·3	30·0
No.	26	7	10	1

[1] Differences between groups were assessed using the t test. $t = 2·22$, $df = 31$, $p = 0·05$.

'With the others the disease was never explained fully and the doctors never said how much attention they needed. They just said, "Don't pamper them," and I often felt if I'd known the whole story of the disease I could have been more understanding to them. The other wee fellows used to bawl and scream and I used to be so cross, and they cried continually. It's awful when you don't know they have an incurable disease that affects them in this way. Had I known I would have had so much more patience—but I didn't know. Now I have more patience with him. [Then, she added,] I'm often puzzled now wondering am I doing enough for him—is there something more I should be doing that I'm not.'

The association between the degree of parental visiting of the sick child in hospital and the parents' change in expectation score

Interestingly, parents who visited their child every day when he was hospitalised tended to change their expectations for him significantly less than parents who visited less often. Of the forty-four sets of parents for whom a corporate expectation change score was available, twenty-two visited their child every day whilst he was hospitalised. Such couples had a mean expectation change score of 7·9. By contrast, the four couples who visited their child only three times a week had a mean expectation change score of 24·7.[1] Similarly, the five couples who visited their sick child only one day a week had a mean expectation change score of 19·2.[2]

This relationship might arise for several reasons. It could be that parents who appreciate the need for daily visiting also appreciate the need for normality in their child's life. By contrast, parents who are less concerned with the child's emotional welfare in hospital, may also find difficulty in recollecting his needs for growth when he returns home. Equally, where parents were unable to visit—either due to their own fears concerning hospital visiting, or because of distance or financial embarrassment—they may try to compensate subsequently by over-protecting the sick child. This was certainly true of some bereaved parents. As mentioned earlier in Chapter 8, some parents who had lost previous children experienced great

[1] The difference between these 2 groups was assessed using the t test. t = 4·69, df = 24, p = 0·01.
[2] This group of parents was compared with the group of parents who visited daily, differences being assessed using the t test. t = 2·56, df = 25, p = 0·05.

emotional distress at the thought of visiting the existing sick child in hospital and several declined to do so because of their fear that this child might also die. Such parents fully appreciated their own limitations in this respect, and may have tried to compensate the child later for their failure to visit.

Relationship between the child's ability to speak of his illness and his parents' change in expectations for him

When children were assessed according to their ability to communicate about their illness in an age-appropriate fashion, it was found that the best communicators came from families which showed least change in expectations. Conversely, the poorest communicators came from families who exhibited the greatest overall change in expectation. Table 26 gives details of the overall expectation change scores of forty-four sets of parents, according to the degree of age-appropriate communication displayed by their sick child.[1]

Table 26 *Mean expectation change score displayed by parents, according to the degree of age-appropriate illness communication exhibited by their sick child*

Degree of communication displayed by sick child	None	Poor	Moderate	Good
Mean expectation change score displayed by parents	16·2	16·2	5·2	7·1
No.	6	15	12	11

[1] Differences between the expectation change scores of parents of 'non' and 'good' child communicators were statistically significant at the 0·05 level, using the t test, t = 2·49, df = 15. Differences between the scores of parents of 'non' and 'moderate' communicators reached statistical significance at the 0·01 level, using the t test, t = 3·60, df = 16. Differences in the expectation change score of parents of 'good' and 'poor' communicators were significant at the 0·05 level, using the t test, t = 2·10, df = 24, and between the 'moderate' and 'poor' communicators at the 0·02 level, using the t test, t = 2·75, df = 25.

11

Sick children

'The four things I'm afraid of are being ill, because I might die next day; being hurt, because I might not get better again; missing school, because I might not get my education—not get good, growing up, because when I'm going to grow up some man might come along and hit me—worst of all is being hurt.'

(Ten-year-old cf boy)

During childhood, the individual develops and masters all the basic physical, intellectual and social skills required for separate adult life. Childhood is therefore a period of intense and often painful learning, during which the growing child needs constant loving encouragement. In this respect, sick and well children have comparable needs, both require a relaxed and sustaining atmosphere in which to grow.

Sadly, however, in contrast to his well brothers and sisters, the sick child's bid for independence may not only be hazarded by his physical limitations, but additionally—and inadvertently—by his parents' attitudes. Challenging and confusing early symptoms, shock and self-doubt accompanying diagnosis, fears attaching to flare-ups of disease, to treatments and hospitalisations, may render it impossible for even the best intentioned parents to relax fully, and enjoy and assist their sick child's self-assertive strivings. In a bid to expiate their own personal feelings of guilt, failure and responsibility, parents may unconsciously alter their child-rearing techniques and their attitudes towards and expectations for the sick child. As a result, they may tend to over-protect and cosset the child, removing him yet further from the normality so essential for personality growth. Indeed, even before birth some chronically sick children may be subjected to a non-normal intra-uterine environment, the mother being emotionally and physically strained.

When one considers the development of any chronically sick child, one must therefore remember that one is assessing behaviour which results not only from the disease but more especially from the whole amalgam of social experiences, hardships, anxieties and evasions which surround it. In charting the fears and anxieties of children in this situation, one is not so much chronicling inevitable concomitants of chronic disease but emphasising the way in which faulty social processes may inadvertently add to the child's handicap. By endeavouring to discover the social factors which are associated with difficulties in the child's development one is therefore illuminating one possible way of preventing or reversing these processes, thereby alleviating some of the distress involved.

With children suffering from cf, there is clear evidence of faulty social processes and a non-normal domestic environment from earliest days; for example, 20 per cent of the group studied were thought to have sustained pronounced emotional and physical stress during their neo-natal period due to maternal knowledge and fear of the disease. An even greater number probably sustained similar intra-uterine stresses attributed by their mothers to general emotional upset or an unsettled domestic environment.

With the exception of the three children whose initial symptoms were sufficient to warrant immediate diagnosis and medical intervention, the early days of most cystic children were clouded by the presence of ephemeral and confusing preliminary symptoms. Understandably, such symptoms distressed parents, making them question their own child-rearing abilities and diminishing their natural joy in the child. Where parents sought medical advice, only to be met by scepticism, personal insecurities and self-doubts were maximised, and this was especially damaging to those who doubted their own powers of perception or instinctive parental skills. As a consequence, therefore, many parents found it hard to maintain that aura of personal optimism so necessary for the satisfactory development of their growing child. Their diminished self-confidence in turn affected both the child's response to them and also his own emergent sense of self. Instead of gradually gaining confidence in his own abilities, feelings of anxiety and self-doubt arose and were accentuated by the galaxy of restraints, inhibitions, and excesses to which he was subjected. Few sick children were handled in the same way as their well brothers and sisters. Almost half were punished less frequently than they deserved, making for tensions between them and their siblings. About a quarter were expected to do less well in terms of either school achievement or participation in physical activities. Almost half the parents admitted that they were not happy with their handling of the child, and parents who were most distressed in this respect, and who exhibited greatest overall change in attitude and behaviour towards the sick child, were parents who had either lost previous children or who were themselves showing signs of severe mental stress. In such families, the child was over-protected to the extent that his separate existence was threatened, a factor resented by children of all ages, but most especially by older children; for example, a fourteen-year-old told me that of all the frustrations he resented, the worst was produced by his mother when 'she brings me in because she's afraid I might get hurt'.

Understandably, parental fears were accentuated by the presence of continuing or dramatic symptoms, such as bowel prolapse. Parents often panicked when faced with such sudden and unexplained occurrences and the child, sensing their anxiety, also became afraid. It was not, therefore, surprising to find that children coping with this symptom exhibited a significantly greater level of fearfulness both in their general behaviour at home and in their protest behaviour when faced with the stresses of hospitalisation.

Similarly, where the sick child required very extensive home-based therapy to counteract his symptoms, he was very quick to appreciate his parents' attitudes towards this. Where they were overwhelmingly positive, he generally complied despite inherent frustrations. Where they were ambivalent, he often played on their insecurities to his own advantage. Where his parents' approach to therapy was negative—either they were ashamed or afraid of the implications—almost invariably his attitude to treatment was also one of shame or fear, and protest behaviour was maximised, or therapy refused. In such cases, the child's negative attitude to treatment was frequently generalised to the illness itself, so that it also became taboo, the child feeling correspondingly demeaned.

Hospitalisation, especially where this was inadequately supported, seemed the greatest challenge to the sick child's developing sense of self-confidence. In hospital, many young children felt abandoned and unlovable, and most protested strongly against such feelings both at the time and afterwards, when they returned to the safety of their home. Even older children who were better able to comprehend the need for hospitalisation often felt frightened or subtly damaged by procedures they sustained.

Erosive self-doubts were accentuated by a general aura of secrecy surrounding the disease. Only 29 per cent of the fifty-eight children I saw had been told the name of their illness, only one child had been told that the disease was inherited, less than one child in ten was prepared in advance for going into hospital, and only 21 per cent of children had been told anything about the way in which the disease affected their body. While, with younger children, this reticence might be understandable, it seemed most inappropriate with older, more questioning children. Despite this, less than a third of the school-age children had parents who had adequately informed them about their illness. Over two-thirds had their questions met with reticence or evasion, despite obvious interest and anxiety on their part. Parents justified this lack of communication by saying that they did not wish to distress the child yet further. Some felt unable to teach the child the facts in the 'right' way, or argued that the child was too young to be bothered, or didn't notice. Whilst one can sympathise with many of these motives, in effect the parents' attitude contributed to the sick child's overall sense of uncertainty and potentiated his feelings of insecurity. For example, a sixteen-year-old boy confided:

> 'If I'm ill, I wonder what is going to happen next. Being ill, you see, you're lying in bed, and it gets worse and worse, and you don't know what is going to happen and you have to get the doctor and wonder what he is going to say.'

Similarly, parents seemed unwilling to face up to the fact that the child might be emotionally affected by his illness state. Only 22 per cent of the fifty-eight children were thought by their parents to pay much attention to their physical symptoms. Equally, only seven were thought to be 'frightened, resentful or sad at being different from others', and only two were thought by their parents to be alarmed at how their illness might affect them in the future. Yet, as I will emphasise later in this chapter, over half the school-age children told me that the illness made them sad, and many openly expressed considerable fears concerning it; for example, a ten-year-old boy said he was afraid of

'being ill, because I might die next day; being hurt, because I might not get better again; missing school, because I might not get my education—not get good, growing up because when I'm going to grow up some man might come along and hit me— worst of all is being hurt'.

Whilst it is understandable that young non-verbal children cannot communicate and thereby gain reassurance for such fears, it was sad to find that older children felt equally unable to confide their anxieties and obtain the necessary emotional and practical support. The majority of school-age children said they had never been able to confide these fears in anyone before. They said their parents 'wouldn't listen' or 'might laugh', or 'they'd be embarrassed'. In this way, as in others, many sick children demonstrated an exaggerated ability to perceive their parents' feeling tone. Similarly, again mirroring their parents' attitudes, very few children felt they could confide in their doctor. Several felt 'it would be too difficult to explain. I wouldn't have the right words'. Yet, where children were able to confide and had their queries met with simple explanations, they seemed less tense and anxious.

Understandably, the innumerable stresses and faulty social processes associated with chronic illness took their toll in terms of the child's general development. Not surprisingly, therefore, most of the children I saw, although quite normal in terms of their motor and intellectual development, displayed problem behaviour throughout childhood.

The pre-school days

During the first months, before diagnosis was made and adequate prophylactic treatment commenced, problems were generally produced by the child's unexplained symptoms. In some cases, babies failed to thrive or make adequate weight gains despite voracious appetites. In other instances, they were sickly, cross, and refused nourishment. Often the mother was faced with frequent bulky, foul-smelling stools. Describing this stage in her baby's life, Mrs C., the wife of a butcher, said:

'Our baby was always pale and black-ringed under his eyes, though we always took him to a baby clinic every week. I blamed it on his food and swapped the food around. We thought it was wind and gave him Nurse Harveys and Milk of Magnesia, but nothing worked. I couldn't take him even to the shops for the smell of his motions in the pram. He woke in the middle of the night, choking. I didn't know what to think, worrying.'

Several other examples of the difficulties encountered during infancy are given above (see p. 27), but two points are worthy of emphasis. First, the infant's pre-diagnostic physical condition frequently precluded the possibility of optimal overall growth, and, second, his symptoms almost invariably aroused anxiety, which, in turn, must have communicated itself to him. Numerous writers have emphasised the way in which parental preoccupation of this sort can adversely affect the development of even the youngest infant (Robertson, 1965; Freud, 1969), and difficulties must have been maximised when the unfortunate parents eventually obtained a diagnosis and sustained the full gamut of shock, grief, physical ill-health, and guilt that followed. In addition, the ailing child was invariably hospitalised for pre-diagnostic testing and many mothers felt that this adversely affected their infant's behaviour—both because of the emotional shock sustained and also because of the changes in routine which took place. In view of these stresses, it was not unexpected to find that, even when adequate prophylactic therapy was commenced, the young child's behaviour continued to be essentially non-normal.

Post-diagnostic problems Table 27 gives details of the post-diagnostic problems displayed by the fifty-eight subject children during the pre-school phase.[1] From this, it is obvious that difficulties were encountered in all the major areas of development. The preponderance of these problems is at least twice that normally occurring in this age range.

---

[1] Interestingly, the study children are similar in this respect to a group of cystic children studied in the east of Scotland (Cull *et al.*, 1972). In Northern Ireland, however, a slightly greater preponderance of problem behaviour was observed. Two possible explanations for this are (1) the high level of pregnancy stress sustained by the study group and (2) the high level of anxiety engendered in the study mothers by their more widespread experience of infant mortality.

Table 27 *Post-diagnostic problems displayed by cystic children during the pre-school phase, as reported by their mothers (%)*

Feeding	56
Toileting	79
Behaviour	59
Sleep disorders	55
No.	58

Post-diagnostic feeding difficulties Virtually half the under-fives had feeding problems at one time or another, ranging from extreme 'peckiness' or a refusal to eat, to the kind of voracious appetite which nightly cleared out the larder, and even sucked the toothpaste from its tube.

Both types of feeding difficulty worried parents. With their newfound knowledge of the child's illness, and their pronounced sense of responsibility for his welfare, parents often measured the child's progress in terms of the normality of his eating habits. If he ate too much and still failed to gain weight, they took it as evidence that the disease was still poorly controlled. Thus, as one mother said:

'I didn't seem to be able to fill her. She was always crying for more. She could take three dinners, not one. She would finish her porridge in three minutes and cry for more, and at a year she could eat half a packet of digestive biscuits and half a swiss roll with a cup of tea. But still she didn't grow. It was desperate.'

Parents of faddy eaters often felt obliged to push food into the reluctant child, fearing that without it he might die. As one mother said: 'He was very small and skinny. Always crying. I used to have to force him to eat—make him take it. I always had to make him take it.' The mother of a four-year-old commented: 'His biggest problem is not eating enough. We have had battles—a lot—trying to get food in.'

Post-diagnostic toileting difficulties Approximately three-quarters of the children displayed toileting difficulties. In 41 per cent of cases, the mother described training as 'difficult', in three cases it was 'stormy'. Even after pot training was accomplished, virtually half the children wet themselves either during the day or at night and about one-third soiled themselves. Occasionally, training was so long delayed that the child was not properly dry or clean until he had been several years at primary school. The majority of mothers coping with these difficulties reported consequent personal upset, confusion and uncertainty. Their self-confidence in the training situation was frequently eroded by their knowledge of the child's illness. They were uncertain as to whether his soiling or wetting was a symptom of the disease, and therefore to be tolerated, or whether it was a gesture of defiance, and therefore to be checked. Rearing methods correspondingly oscillated between indulgence and reproval, making for even greater difficulties all round.

As mentioned above (see p. 114), parents and children coping with sudden bowel prolapse were especially disadvantaged in this respect. Many were too frightened of possible recurrence to insist too rigidly on regular pot training.

In addition, 40 per cent of mothers found the smell of their child's motions unpleasant, complaining that it pervaded the house, producing shame on their part. The mother of a three-year-old expressed her feelings thus: 'At the beginning it was awful. If anyone comes to the door when he's in, it is embarrassing. It's a very powerful smell for strangers.' Young children were hidden away to have their nappies changed, and air fresheners were much in evidence. Even very young children came to appreciate the need for these; for example, a two-year-old demanded, 'Mummy, spray,' or, 'Mummy, hold nose' when on the pot. In a few extreme cases, parental disturbance was such that the children were refused permission to use the toilet when visitors were around. Understandably, this attitude affected the child's view of himself and his relationship with his parents; for example, one seven-year-old boy said his mother annoyed him most when 'I want something and she won't give it to me—like being allowed into the toilet when the visitors are coming.'

Occasionally, it was not the parents' sense of shame, but rather the distaste displayed by family friends, which made for difficulties; for example, the mother of a five-year-old confided:

'She has never ever said she was embarrassed, but once she was in a car and she smelt, and people opened windows and made remarks, and then got a bucket of water to wash out the car and it upset her and she noticed. We never let her in a car again . . . we don't go out so often with her now, she gets embarrassed.'

The mother of a small boy said:

'He doesn't like to smell. He says someone else has done it. He said all the wee boys said it was him and he said it wasn't. Up until a couple of years ago he really didn't know it was him smelling. He said it wasn't. But now he knows.'

As a consequence, some pre-school children were thought to avoid the toilet voluntarily when others were around, and this avoidance was especially true of older children, many of whom would not use school toilets for fear of rebuffs. One may conjecture that in this, as in other ways, a general attitude of shame was quickly conveyed to the child, negatively colouring his own opinion of himself, and accentuating any inherent physical difficulties in accomplishing bowel control.

Problem behaviours not associated with the illness   Over half the pre-school children showed evidence of problem behaviours not directly associated with the illness. Most usually, these took the form of excessive temper tantrums and inordinately demanding behaviour. Even minor changes in the domestic environment were reacted to adversely and parents learnt to modify their behaviour accordingly. Some children exhibited ultra-dependent behaviour, trying to monopolise the mother's entire attention and becoming jealous of brothers and sisters. Such behaviour was manifested by clinging onto the mother during the day and endeavouring to secure her attention at night. In extreme cases, this became very distressing for the mother; for instance, the mother of a five-year-old boy described him as 'demanding, tearful, difficult and jealous'. She continued: 'He's not happy in any way. He feels himself an outcast. He used to be crying all night wanting to be picked up, and he's at it yet. I can't even open my mouth to him or he starts to cry. He's just like a big baby.' Another mother said of her four-year-old: 'She used to get into terrible tempers. She used to bite her brother regularly. She bit right through his coat. I used to worry what she would do to the other children in the street. She would throw things at him, kick him even yet.' The mother of another pre-schooler confided: 'I have to do a lot of settling up because she really would go on and on about things. Sometimes she really upsets me with her quarrelling. She goes on and on, and I feel like having a wee cry with frustration.'

In this context, it would seem essential to remember the high degree of hospitalisation which this group sustained. Many of the behaviour difficulties encountered at home by parents may be attributed more properly to insecurities following hospitalisation rather than behaviour difficulties related only to the illness. Often, jealousies and ultra-dependency seemed to stem from fear of abandonment, the child fearing to go off on his own, or to have his mother parted from him. Thus, 'if he knew I was going out or doing something he would play me up' and 'the other day my mother was minding him, and he said, "Will my Mummy ever come back?" He does say that from time to time.'

Sleep difficulties in pre-school children   Fears of abandonment may also underlie the problems connected with sleep or getting to sleep experienced by over half the pre-school children. Forty-five per cent of the study group were thought by their parents to have woken regularly during the night, 39 per cent to have taken more than half an hour to fall asleep, 30 per cent to have nightmares, and 21 per cent to be fearful at bed time. Sometimes children seemed afraid to actually lose consciousness; for example, a four-year-old was described as 'yelling and screaming as if he was emotionally upset.' A two-year-old was given to 'shouting out in his sleep at night. He is very restless. He could be in pain or it could be a nightmare. It's difficult to say. He sits up in bed with his hands out. He's at an age when he can't say.' Older children complained of frightening dreams, such as monsters coming to take them away, or losing themselves a long distance from home. Not unexpectedly, some children endeavoured to protract bedtime. Thus: 'He wants a story read to him. He prolongs his good nights as long as possible. He comes down after we put him to bed.'

Many parents empathetically relaxed their normal stringency over bedtime and developed the habit of bringing the young child down for a talk, an extra cuddle or a drink. Many of the children demanded, and 56 per cent of the parents permitted the child, to sleep with them in their bed, either occasionally or, in a few cases, every night. The oldest child who regularly shared his parents' bed was ten. Sometimes bed-sharing became a joke between the married partners; for example, one father told me with a chuckle: 'We don't need family planning with Barbara in our bed.' More often, it was regarded with slight disquiet; for example, one mother commented: 'He gets up most nights and wanders in. He curls up beside me. He only wants beside me.' Then she added, with slight annoyance: 'When I had to go to hospital myself he didn't do it. He wouldn't make any attempt to join his father.' Another mother, whose daughter 'would never dream of sleeping on her own', took the child to the family doctor who said: 'I don't sympathise with you. It's your own fault. She's making a prisoner of you. It won't do her any harm to cry.' She commented: 'He was right too.'

Social development of pre-school children   All the twenty-eight pre-school children were assessed in terms of their social development using the Vineland Social Maturity Scale. The average social development score was 103, and the range and scatter were normal, being evenly distributed from 75 to 138. In certain developmental areas, such as self-help, some children were slightly behind the level expected for their chronological age and this slight retardation is probably due to the excessive concern of parents for their welfare. By protecting and cosseting the child, rather than making him do small jobs for himself, some mothers obviously felt they could minimise self-blame if anything went wrong in the future. Occasionally, it was also obvious that, as with other handicapped children (Gibbons, 1974), the mothers of pre-school cystic children were genuinely uncertain as to what they could legitimately expect of the sick child in terms of self-help. Whereas most parents are aware of the culturally determined developmental goals for normal children and encourage their well children to attain these, parents of sick children are often at a loss to know to what standards their sick children should be expected to conform. Their confusion in this respect is mirrored in their comments. For example, the mother of a four-year-old, speaking of her need to settle his quarrels, said: 'He comes to me no matter how simple they are. I wonder if I'm making a real softie of him—over-doing it—but I couldn't bear to let him cry over it.'

Going to school

Not unexpectedly, in view of the preponderance of pre-school problem behaviour, many parents anticipated problems in terms of settling their sick child into the school community. Many thought that the dependent behaviour seen at home would be exaggerated, and some expected tearful, clinging farewells. Surprisingly, this was not the case. Of the thirty study children who were attending school, only 26 per cent had any problems settling in and only 20 per cent were thought by their parents to have subsequently experienced problems in going to school. The child's usual response was one of enthusiasm, as evidenced by these comments: 'She had no problems whatsoever. That was the most amazing thing to me. I was dreading leaving her, but the teacher came along and put her hand out and she took it and off she went.' 'I had more problems when he first went than he did. I cried to dinner time, but he didn't.' 'It surprised me how well she settled. She was so glad to get in with the other children—especially the little girls of her own age—she was fascinated by them.' Many parents were clearly most relieved by the normality of this occurrence. Equal relief was produced by the fact that the child's intially positive attitude to school appeared to persist. Up to the time of the survey, only 26 per cent of children were thought ever to have been 'clingy or worried about leaving' their mother, only 16 per cent were thought to have been 'sick before leaving for school', only 23 per cent dawdled or invented reasons for staying away or 'complained of the children', and only 16 per cent 'complained that the work was too hard'. The majority of children seemed to accept their new role and environment with alacrity, tried very hard to succeed and, if poor health kept them away, almost fought with their parents to be allowed to go. In this way, parents often commented that the attitude of their sick child to school was better than that of their other well children. As one mother of an eight-year-old expressed it: 'She's definitely different. Everything has to be done properly—that's her best. Everything has to be right.'

The sick child's surprisingly positive response to school may occur for several reasons. First, going to school may reassure him concerning his normality, and, should he have questioned this, it might relieve him of some underlying anxiety. Second, school might present him with a more challenging environment than home, enabling him to try out all manner of nascent skills unhindered by parental over-protection. In this way, the sick child might view school as a chance to prove his ability in a freer environment. Finally, in order to compensate for any 'lack' or sense of 'difference', which he might have experienced during his pre-school days, the child's normal age-appropriate wish to conform might be accentuated, thereby becoming an adaptive mechanism enabling him to overcome personal feelings of inadequacy.

Basic intelligence and academic attainment   The basic intelligence level of all school-age children was assessed using the Wechsler Intelligence Scale for Children. Test results indicated that study children were quite normal in terms of their intellectual development. The mean IQ was 104 and the range and scatter were well within the limits of normality, being from 72 to 137.

Testing revealed that 50 per cent of the girls and 37 per cent of the boys scored significantly better on the vocabulary subtest than on any other IQ Scale item. This finding adds some credence to Lawler's observations concerning the heightened conversational abilities of cystic children (Lawler *et al.,* 1966), and the possibility that conversational skills are used adaptively by the child to win approval and allay anxiety will be discussed later in this chapter.

In addition, to establish his competence in basic school work, each child was given three standard attainment tests—the Schonell Reading Test, the Schonell Spelling Test and the Vernon Arithmetic-Mathematics Test. In view of the apparent intellectual normality of the children, it was presumed that they would achieve an age-appropriate standard of attainment in these skills. But this was not so. Even when standards were adjusted to accord with mental age (based on chronological age and IQ), all but one of the cystic children were retarded in one or more subject. Interestingly, the exception was an adopted child whose parents, when interviewed, knew nothing about the disease except that the child needed replacement enzymes in order to grow. Fortunately, this boy was only slightly affected by the illness and remained in good health, needing no hospitalisation and only occasional check-ups in the outpatient clinic. He was therefore reared as a normal child.

Fifty-five per cent of the boys and 66 per cent of the girls were retarded in two or more basic school subjects to the extent that their test scores were twelve months or more behind those expected of children of their age and intelligence. Obviously, this degree of retardation must have affected their ability to keep up with their age mates and must have created further insecurities for them in the classroom.

In this respect, it was interesting to compare the attainments of cystic children attending a special school for delicate children with those attending normal school. One argument that is often advanced to support attendance at a special school is the argument that delicate children progress better when they feel protected, and do not have to compete with healthy children. Clearly, the limited scope of this study does not permit extensive comment on this point. However, it was interesting to find that there was no real difference in attainment between children attending a special school for delicate children and those coping with the rough and tumble of well peers. The total average retardation for special school children in three subjects was thirty-five months behind the standard expected of their age and ability as compared with an average total retardation of thirty-four months for children attending normal school.

Even children who were only slightly affected by their symptoms, and able to attend school regularly, were found to be as retarded in basic school work as children in poorer physical health.

Retardation in basic school work associated with anxiety   Why does this retardation occur? One possibility is that the study children, despite their enthusiasm to be in school, were basically too anxious about their social acceptability and essential security to really pay attention to school work. This seemed especially true of older children, some of whom had difficulty in concentrating; for example, an eleven-year-old was described as 'a very unsettled pupil. He can't sit in a chair. He walks around.' Ever-present illness symptoms, such as cough and wind, contributed to the child's anxiety, eliciting teasing or ostracism in class. In addition, the constant need for replacement enzymes before school lunch contributed to embarrassment, so that often, with increasing age, the child resorted to evasive behaviour, getting out of class early and swallowing capsules in the toilet, or occasionally throwing them away.

Two factors were found to relate to retardation:

(1) the sick child's overall level of anxiety, as measured by the Taylor Manifest Anxiety Scale. Children who were retarded in two subjects had higher scores on the TMAS than children who were retarded in only one subject.*[1]

* Differences between groups were assessed using the t test.

[1] $t = 2.90$, df $= 7$, $p < 0.05$.

(2) the cf child's general response to school. Children who exhibited problem behaviour in school were most retarded.[*][1]

Clearly, the happiest, most settled children progressed best in terms of basic school work. Conversely, those with problems in other areas did least well in academic work.

Retardation in basic school work fostered by over-protective attitudes
Retardation might also result from the fact that for many parents the child's health was of more importance than his academic achievements and consequently school work was not their most crucial concern. Twenty-five per cent of the ninety-seven parents interviewed said that they actually expected less of their child in terms of school achievement because of the illness. This attitude must undoubtedly have conveyed itself to the children who thereby adjusted their own expectations accordingly. Similarly, some teachers may have reduced their standards out of 'concern' for the child; for example, one mother was told by her son's class teacher: 'I hope he's not working too hard.' This mother commented: 'Perhaps she felt she shouldn't let him do too much.' Similarly, another mother described her child's teachers as 'very good to her'. She added: 'They know she's not well, and they treat her as something special.' Occasionally, this attitude was so obvious that even the child and his friends remarked on it; for instance, one six-year-old was asked by his pals: 'Why don't you ever get slapped—even if your name is on the blackboard?' This sensitive child then felt forced to pretend that he was being regularly slapped. His mother commented: 'At one time, I was so worried I was ready to go up to the school and complain, then he admitted he was pretending.' This would seem to be another instance of the child's social environment inadvertently adding to his handicap.

The social adjustment of school-age cf children, as seen in school
Inevitably, the stressful experiences to which cf children were subjected and the changes in parental attitudes and social environment affected their social behaviour. When compared with a carefully matched control group and assessed objectively by their class teachers using a Bristol Social Adjustment Guide, cf children were found to be significantly more unsettled, especially in the

*Differences between groups were assessed using the t test.
[1] $t = 2.17$, df $= 29$, $p < 0.05$.

realms of unforthcomingness and under-reactivity.*[1] This was especially true of children with severe symptoms. Indeed, such under-reactivity would seem characteristic of many chronically ill children, being observed in some chronically ill members of the control group in this study and emerging as a characteristic of asthmatic children, studied previously by me (Burton, 1968). In this respect, sick children seem to develop a special and understandable defensiveness in order to ward off occurrences which might prove stressful for them.

The unforthcoming and under-reactive child is afraid of 'new tasks and strange situations, and is timid with people, while maintaining a need for affection' (Stott, 1958). His timidity is apparent both in his contacts with staff and fellow pupils. He shrinks from *active* involvement with either, yet seems interested in both. Unforthcoming children are often so quiet that it is hard to know whether they are participating in classwork. When faced with new and challenging tasks they seem unwilling or afraid to begin and need great encouragement to take part. Understandably, this may affect their formal learning and Stott and Sykes (1956) have concluded that 'as a relief from anxiety about school learning' the unforthcoming child 'may accept the role of being "dull"'. Such defensiveness may further contribute to the observed retardation of study children. To spare themselves the stress of competing, sick children often opt out scholastically and are content to let others win the accolades.

Similarly, in terms of physical activity and play, the unforthcoming child may shrink from any active involvement and prefer to wander off alone or engage in some solitary pastime. In this respect, sick boys seem most ill-at-ease and most timid, perhaps because when faced with normal boyish rowdy play they feel most disadvantaged. Some give reasons to justify their reserve; for example: 'I might fall,' or 'They'd want to play tigers.' Others can give no reason: 'Just it scares me, it frightens me. I don't know why. I just don't like it.'

Children with cf fear physical violence, both the scrapping of other children and being slapped by teachers. They also fear verbal abuse and seem to guard themselves against being involved in either by behaving as correctly and meekly as possible: 'I wouldn't like to

* Differences between groups were assessed using the t test.

[1] $t = 2.6323$, df $= 38$, $p < 0.05$.

get slapped. I'm afraid of getting slapped. One teacher, she slapped everybody for no reason. That wasn't fair, sure it wasn't?' (ten-year-old). 'When they're talking, the teacher has to hit them, and I hate watching them getting smacked. I don't like watching it' (eight-year-old). 'When somebody else is shouting, you get smacked and all' (seven-year-old).

Perhaps such 'good' behaviour subserves two useful functions: first, it prevents the sick child from being involved in situtations which might prove physically stressful for him, and, second, it affirms his acceptability in the eyes of others despite physical symptoms and medicaments which cause him so much embarrassment.

Five symptoms of social unsettledness (contained in the Bristol Social Adjustment Guide) were specific to chronically ill children—both subject children suffering from cf, and their chronically ill controls—but were never once used to describe well children. They were: (UB_1, paying attention in class) 'So quiet you don't really know if he's following or not'; (RB_2, informal play) 'Has his own special solitary activity'; (UA_6, liking for sympathy) 'Likes sympathy but is reluctant to ask'; (UB_3, team games) 'Has to be encouraged to take part'; (UB_7, classroom behaviour) 'Too timid to be any trouble'.

Seventy per cent of the cystic children in this study exhibited one or more of those symptoms. Some displayed them all. In this respect, as previously mentioned, the study children were significantly different from the control children.*[1]

School problems related to predisposing factors When a global assessment was made of the child's response to school, as witnessed by both his teacher and his mother, some children were found to be markedly more problematic than others. Generally, such problem children were:

(1) older children. The mean age of children with school problems was significantly higher than that of non-problematic children.[2]

---

[1] In this respect, Northern Irish children closely resembled a similar group of cystic children studied in the east of Scotland (Cull *et al.*, 1972), though Northern Irish children showed a slightly higher preponderance of unforthcomingness. This could be due to the more anxious nature of their domestic environment, in turn due to the higher mortality rate in the Northern Irish sample.

* Differences between groups assessed using the t test.

[2] $t = 2.14$, df $= 29$. $p < 0.05$.

(2) children in poorer health. Children with school problems had poorer ratings on the McCrae Scale than children without school problems.*[1]

(3) children showing greater response to their illness. Children with school problems tended to show more response to their illness, as assessed by their parents, than children without school problems.[2]

In addition, as mentioned previously, children with school problems tended to be more retarded in basic school work than happier, less problematic children.

One is forced therefore to conclude that, even within a group of school-age sick children, there are considerable individual differences in terms of settledness. Whilst some appear to show little response to the illness at home or in school, others, either due to increasing age, heightened sensitivity or poorer physical health, exhibit considerable unhappiness and benefit least from formal education.

Social unsettledness displayed at home

Even away from school, in their safe and non-stressful home environment, many school-age cystic children were timid. Dependent habits, formed early, continued; for example, a mother who had newly returned to work said of her six-year-old daughter: 'She resents the fact that I work, not that it changes her life in any way, but she resents it. She doesn't like the fact that I do anything outside the house.' Similarly, fears regarding abandonment persisted. The mother of a seven-year-old said: 'She's worried in case I go away and don't come back. Who will look after her if I don't come back. She can't bear it if I'm not around.' New fears were also apparent—some connected with school; thus the mother of a nine-year-old boy observed: 'If something happened about his homework he would get into a tizzy. "I have to, Mummy, I have to," he would say if he needed something for his homework and there was no way of getting it.' In the same way, sleep problems persisted. Often the older child was sufficiently self-controlled to replace his earlier nightly prowlings with more restrained, though slightly anxious, inquiries, such as: 'Will you be coming up soon?' In a few cases, however, night fears seemed to increase with increasing age, the child

*Differences between groups were assessed using the t test.
[1] $t = 2.64$, df $= 24$, $p < 0.05$.
[2] $t = 2.97$, df $= 29$, $p < 0.01$.

appearing to use fear of sleep as an excuse for reassurance concerning wider—though often unspecified—fears; for instance, a nine-year-old girl who refused to discuss or recognise her illness was described by her mother as

> 'a strange little girl. She goes to bed at nine and she starts to worry about her homework, or, if she's going somewhere, she starts to worry about these things. She's in tears about it every night. She worries about silly things, something she has to do next day—a wee period of worrying every night.'

The sick child's approach to play

Timidity was also apparent in the sick child's approach to play. Seventy-three per cent of boys and 76 per cent of girls preferred to play at home, close to the comforting presence of their parents. This attitude undoubtedly mirrored that of the parents for whom play outside the home often became synonymous with infection, danger, or damage. Three mothers, typical of many, described their feelings in this matter: 'I'm frightened that other children might hit her. I'm always scared. There's nothing behind her. She's like a fly.' 'He would go into other houses but I prefer not to let him for other houses are not so clean. This house is clean.' 'I tend to protect her in that way in case the other children bully her. I'm always apprehensive in case she is bullied.' Very occasionally, protective attitudes were generalised to embrace all the children in the family, including the well children. Thus one mother confided: 'I never allow the children out to play. I suppose because we have only two OK and no more to come. I would never let anything happen to them.' This form of over-protection was most pronounced in families who had lost previous children, and is discussed in greater detail above (see p. 153).

The sick child's response to his illness

Parents were asked to evaluate the way in which their child responded to his illness. Table 28 gives details of the responses obtained to a series of questions devised to elicit information concerning this topic. Generally, pre-school children were thought by their parents to be oblivious to their illness, though a few such children were thought to gain special pleasure from the additional attention they

Table 28 *The reactions of cystic children to their illness, as assessed by their parents*

Reaction of sick child to the illness	Pre-school children (%)	School-age children (%)	Total group (%)
Child alarmed at how illness might affect him in the future	0	6	3·5
Child pleased at getting special attention	28	43	36
Child pays undue attention to physical symptoms	7	36	22
Child self-conscious or worried about reactions of others to the illness	3	47	27
Child frightened, resentful or sad at being different from others	0	23	12
Child worried about his physical appearance	0	40	20
No.	28	30	58

received. This response became more apparent with increasing age, and 43 per cent of the over-fives were thought to enjoy the attention provided by the illness, occasionally even to the point of hypochrondriasis. Thus, one ten-year-old was thought to 'love dentists. He really looks forward to it. He loves going to hospital for tests as long as he doesn't have to stay. He loves to lie in bed at home.' But such hypochrondriasis was the exception rather than the rule. Most children were thought not to like illness experiences, though they traded on the spoiling which acompanied them. The mother of a seven-year-old described it this way: 'He likes a lot of attention. He's not jealous, just demanding—probably because he's always got so much attention. He takes it for granted. He's very attached to me, very dependent.' A six-year-old girl 'likes to be spoilt. She knows she's spoilt because she's delicate. She says, "You've got to be nice to me. I'm delicate. I go to a special school. I'm delicate."'

With increasing age, there was a tendency for the child to become more 'self-conscious or worried about the reactions of others to the illness', and to worry about his physical appearance. Sometimes self-consciousness or fear of physical unacceptability or inadequacy was exhibited by a refusal to undress for PT, clinic visits or when buying new clothes. In the study setting, it was revealed in the drawings children made of themselves and in the disparaging remarks they made concerning these. For example, a seven-year-old girl exhibited her anxiety by heavily shading in the chest area of her self-portrait, sadly commenting, 'I think I'll look like an elephant when I'm finished,' and then later, 'I don't think I'm nice looking at all.' Such fears of bodily inadequacy were most marked in the older, pre-teenage children. Then, for the first time, the child really looked to the future and wondered whether he would be able to cope physically with the strains of holding down a job.

Self-consciousness and physical fears had their roots both in the child's growing appreciation of his physical limitations and also in the unkind comments of siblings and peers. Having to take medicines in public, coughing during physical exertions, being sick unexpectedly, or being noticeably thin and small all proved sources of embarrassment for the growing child. Several children became increasingly self-conscious after being measured publicly in class as part of a New Mathematics project. The mother of a six-year-old said, 'They said in school he was small for his age—that worried him. I asked who was saying it and he said they all were.' Another boy, whose teeth were permanently blackened by antibiotics, was asked, 'What do you clean your teeth with—muck?' He asked his mother, 'Do you think if I kept cleaning my teeth, they would get nice and white?' Many children in poorer physical health found difficulty in keeping up with street play—perhaps one further reason why so many preferred to play at home. Thus the mother of a seven-year-old said:

'He is now starting to feel that he's not able to keep up with the other boys in the street. He would like to keep up with his friends, but he goes with slower boys now. He hangs about a bit. He never says anything, just goes with younger boys now—whereas he used to go with his own age.'

In much the same way, older children were increasingly aware of and preoccupied by their physical symptoms, and 23 per cent were thought to have reached the stage where they had become 'frightened, resentful or sad at being different from others'. Being kept in on wet and cold days contributed to feelings of sadness, and older children became resentful of the fact that they had to have daily therapy whereas others did not require it; for instance, a nine-year-old refused her medicine, saying: 'I'm not going to take this any more. They're not taking it.' Feelings of difference contributed to feelings of shame, despite the parents' attempts to avert this; for example, an eight-year-old forbade her mother to talk of her illness when people inquired about her. 'I said, "Why not? There's nothing to be ashamed of. Everyone has something wrong with them," and she said, "What's wrong with you then?"'

Although few children were reported to be 'alarmed at how the illness might affect them in the future', many children had reached the point of considering the possibility of death. Usually, such thoughts were prompted by the unkind comments of age mates or brothers and sisters; for instance, the mother of a six-year-old told me: 'One wee boy told him in hospital the other day that he'd cf, and the muscles in his back would all go hard and it would go up to his brain and his mind would go away and he'd die, and he cried about that.' Similarly, a five-year-old heard a visitor say, 'These children die before they become teenagers.' Her mother reported: 'She couldn't get it out of her mind. She kept saying, "I'm not going to die. He's not going to make me die. I'll die in my own time."' The youngest child to express a fear of death was two years old.

Parents may be unable to objectively estimate the extent to which their child is affected emotionally by his illness. Understandably, they are often unwilling to admit that it can have emotional consequences. Coping as they do with all the onerous practicalities of his daily care, many have little energy left for worrying about further, more nebulous concerns. This was illustrated by the fact that when parents were asked what, in their estimate, was the child's greatest handicap from his point of view, most parents simply mentioned the necessity to take medicine, or a physical symptom which impeded play, without considering the implications of these in terms of the child's emotional and social development. Only one parent stressed the fact that these things contributed to a feeling of insecurity in the child so that he had himself begun to worry about his future.

Perhaps parents are limited in their ability to comprehend the child's feelings because of the general aura of silence concerning the disease. As mentioned earlier, only 32 per cent of the school-age children in this study felt able to talk over their illness worries with anyone. The others felt their parents would be too embarrassed to listen. In part, their reticence may spring from their heightened sensitivity to others—many cystic children were thought to be exceptionally sympathetic. In part, it may arise from a genuine unwillingness on the part of the parent to discuss the disease with the child. Yet, when the subject was broached sympathetically cystic children were glad to speak of their feelings in this matter, and in conversation 65 per cent of the school-age children expressed a fear of being hurt, 50 per cent of being ill, 47 per cent of going into hospital; 58 per cent of the children said the illness made them sad and 36 per cent said it worried them. Comments such as the following were typical: 'I keep getting these colds. I keep thinking, 'Why am I not like other children?' I can't go out all the time' (ten-year-old). 'I hate getting tired—on a warm day it's the worst. If I run a lot I get puffed and if I do heavy work I get tired. Then I won't be fit for anything and I have to lie down on a stretcher and that gets me worried' (sixteen-year-old). 'If I get out with my friends it eases the worry. If I get out it's better. If I sit here there's worry on my mind but if I go out and have a laugh I don't worry any more' (fifteen-year-old). 'I feel annoyed with it—it depresses me. It makes me sad at home. I want to get out' (eleven-year-old).

While younger children railed against the limitation of their freedom implicit in the need to stay close to the home, older children expressed a fear of physical inadequacy and an apprehension concerning possible unemployment. More sensitive parents perceived this from the child's chance remarks; for example, the mother of a fifteen-year-old said: 'He worries about what he'll do when he grows up and what sort of job he'll get.' The mother of an eleven-year-old found him 'more tense lately. More anxious about the future and what he will do. I don't know why he's so worried about what he's going to do. He was never tense as a child, and I'm not putting any pressure on him about the future or what he will be.' An intelligent seven-year-old even confounded her parents by saying: 'I'm tired being sick. I want to go to Heaven. I told God last night that I want to go to Heaven as a little girl, not to grow up.'

Fears engendered by illness, revealed in a personality test

Generally, fears engendered by the illness and the therapeutic regime seemed well contained by the children concerned. Most were at the level of nagging apprehensions rather than obsessions.

However, it is true to say that by contrast to a control group of children chosen from the same schools, the study children were significantly more anxious concerning their physical safety. When the two groups were compared using six cards taken from the Thematic Apperception Test,[1] cystic children displayed significantly more fear of being hurt, being sick, going into hospital and dying. Their stories were significantly sadder in feeling tone than those of the control children.[2]

A gradual evolution of fears with age was revealed in the stories made up by study children. Unequivocal fears of sickness, death and hospital figure largely in the stories recounted by under-eights, whereas slightly older children display more subtle fears concerning personal inadequacy and unworthiness. There is a gradually increasing awareness that something is wrong, though the reason for this is rarely known. Older children fear that they will be unable to assert themselves, and many wonder how they will cope with work. At all ages there is an obvious fear of loneliness. The following stories, made up by children of different ages, illustrate these points. The first four stories were told to me by a five-year-old and well illustrate the fear of hurt and hospitalisation obvious in this age group.

(3G) 'A woman—she's hurt her eye. She's going to go to the hospital and before it comes off she's got to get it sewn on again.'

(7G) 'A nurse and a wee girl holding a baby. They've hurt themselves—they're at the hospital and I think the man is saying, "You'll have to stay in."'

(3BM) 'A man and he's hurt himself and he's going to go to the hospital and I think he's going to stay in. He'll have to get injections before he gets home. He's thinking about going to hospital and what they're going to do to him and he's thinking they're going to put a bandage on him.'

[1] The Thematic Apperception Test was devised by Morgan and Murray in 1935. This test, used with both adults and children consists of thirty pictures, the majority of which depict life situations involving one or more persons. The subject is asked to make up a story about the picture, and about the people in it. He is invited to discuss their needs, feelings and experiences. It is hoped that he will project his own emotions and preoccupations into these fantasy productions, and any consistency of response from story to story is noted as being a possible indication of the subject's own problems.

[2] Differences between the scores obtained by the two groups were analysed using a one-tailed Wilcoxon Matched-Pairs Signed-Ranks Test. All differences attained a 0·001 level of significance.

(17GF) 'They're going to kill him and that's his Daddy and they're going to kill him and he's going to cry.'

Death is not always clearly understood by younger children, and their resultant confusion and fear are clearly revealed in the following two stories made up by a six-year-old:

(3BM) 'He's dead. The man's dead, and he's up there, down in the bunks that one. He has boots. He's dead. To be dead you're deaf, you're blind, your brain dies—the rest is all right. . . . He's not thinking of anything, he's just dead.'

(8BM) 'There's a boy—that's a man and that. He's dead—a rifle. He's deaf. He's blind and his bare skin. His moustache. His nose. A knife and it cut into there, and a rifle and a boy. He's going to be dead.'

Even young children expressed resentment at the frustrations imposed upon them by their illness; for example, the next story recounted by a six-year-old illustrates his longing to get out to play. This same boy told me in conversation that his biggest fear was of missing school 'because I can get out to play sometimes if I'm at school'.

(13B) 'A boy—he's thinking of going out. He wants to go out to play. He's no socks and shoes. He's sitting down. He wants to go out to play and he's not allowed out. That's why he wants to run out without his socks and shoes. He can't go because his mother doesn't allow him. He's thinking of running out. He's sitting, but I suppose he'll run out.'

Similarly, a seven-year-old recounted this story:

(13B) 'I wish I could go out to play. He's thinking that. Because he's not allowed out, because it's raining.'

Feelings of being singled out or prevented from joining in normal play activities undoubtedly contributed to a growing sense of loneliness amongst the children. The following two stories told by a ten-year-old express this:

(13B) 'The wee boy was very lonely, and he had no one to play with and he was bored and he sat down on the doorstep and he was bored and he had nothing to do. He can see no children playing and he had no bicycle. He might start a fight with another boy or throw stones at a dog, or smash a window with a stone. He might run away from home and take some food with him as well as clothes. His mother might hit him very hard.'

(3BM) 'This wee boy had no one to play with and he smashed the window and his mother beat him. He was crying and he was very lonely and had nothing to do—only play with his gun. He was going to run away from his mother and not come back and take some biscuits and food and lemonade.'

Increasing uncertainty concerning the future, and fears of physical frailty contribute to the need for companionship, and in teenage children this seems especially acute. The final three stories, drawn from a sixteen-year-old's protocol, illustrate this:

(13B) 'In this picture the young boy is lonely and it's an old shack that he lives in. His parents are not rich. He is not well dressed and he has no shoes or stockings on. The house in which he lives looks bare and empty. I think he would be thinking that he would like to live with other people so that he could have friends to play with, to talk with.'

(3GF) 'In this picture you see a woman who looks to be in sorrow. She looks to be a very worried person. If she is worried then she would be very nervous. She's standing there as if she doesn't know what is the matter with her. She looks very tired-looking. She would like to have someone to talk to, to have friends to go out with and enjoy themselves—go to parties and try and get rid of most of the worries, or even to the pictures with a boy friend.'

(16) 'In this picture you see an old man fishing—the place he is fishing is in a very large lake—the reason why he is fishing is because he is lonely or has no one to talk to in the home. He could be living by himself. Fishing is a great sport. It helps you to concentrate on your work and it could take your mind off your worries. Old people live by themselves and they would be afraid of intruders, that they could not stand up against them, and they could be afraid they would be badly hurt, and if they live by themselves and if they were sick they could not send for a doctor and they would have to do everything by themselves—do the housework by themselves and the shopping.'

Children showing most response to their illness

Whilst most children, especially older children, showed some slight response to their illness, there were considerable individual differences in this respect, some children showing very pronounced negative reactions. Such children tended to be:

(1) fearful children of any age. Children who were described by

their mothers as being 'moderately fearful' on the basis of their behaviour at home tended to show significantly more response to their illness than children described by their mothers as 'showing very little fear' in the domestic environment.*[1] Similarly, school-age children who were thought to show a moderate response to their illness had higher ratings on the Taylor Manifest Anxiety Scale than children who were showing only a slight response to their illness.[2]

(2) children who had sustained most hospitalisation. Children who showed no response to their illness had been in hospital significantly less than children who showed either a slight,*[3] moderate,[4] or marked[5] response to their illness. One must admit that these relationships may reflect an age bias, younger children lacking sufficient sensitivity to show a marked response to the illness, and having less chance of being hospitalised, by contrast to older children, for whom the reverse was true.

Children with school problems

As mentioned above (p. 174), children with school problems tended to show more response to their illness than children without school problems. In turn, they tended to be older children in poorer health.

On the basis of these associations, one may conclude that some children seem fearful from earliest days, and these children show the most marked response to their illness. In the pre-school days, this fearfulness is apparent in the children's social contacts and play and in their marked response to stressful happenings such as hospitalisations. Later, fearfulness is apparent in their attitude to school, their behaviour whilst there, and is revealed in the scores they obtain on an objective anxiety scale.

Children showing most fear

The children who were described by their mothers as 'very fearful' or 'moderately fearful', on the basis of their behaviour at home, tended to be:

* Differences between groups were assessed using the t test.

[1] $t = 2.69$, df $= 52$, $p < 0.01$.
[2] $t = 2.35$, df $= 13$, $p < 0.05$.

* Differences between these four groups were assessed using the t test.

[3] $t = 2.58$, df $= 36$, $p < 0.05$.
[4] $t = 3.19$, df $= 35$, $p < 0.01$.
[5] $t = 2.98$, df $= 25$, $p < 0.01$.

(1) Children in poorer health. Fearful children tended to have poorer ratings on the McCrae Rating Scale for chest involvement. In addition, children with rectal prolapse—most often children in poorer general health—were significantly more fearful than children who were not troubled by this symptom.*[1]

(2) Those who showed most response to their illness (as outlined above, p. 182).

(3) Those who protested most in hospital. Children who protested most in hospital were significantly more fearful than children who did not protest at all.[2]

Compensating devices for feared inadequacies

As mentioned earlier in this chapter, children with cf fear physical violence, both the rough and tumble of their peers and chastisement by the teacher. They also fear verbal abuse. Whilst fear of violence is understandable in terms of the child's need to guard himself against experiences which might prove physically overwhelming, fear of verbal abuse cannot be so construed. Yet many sick children lay emphasis on this when describing happenings which they dislike: 'The other children are bad. They talk too much. They talk about everything.' 'I hate them when they say bad words or shout.' 'Sometimes their shouting deafens me.' 'One of them is very rude—he says rude things to everyone.'

It would seem probable that sick children fear the possibility of being inadvertently involved in such debates, and thereby punished or ostracised. By trying to keep outside such fracas the sick child seems to protect himself from physical harm, and also remains as acceptable as possible despite physical symptoms and inadequacies which cause him so much embarrassment. By being 'good', he is trying to gain approval and thereby avoid prejudicing his relationships.

Similarly, many sick children appear to compensate for their supposed physical inadequacies by taking extra care with their dress and appearance. Sometimes such behaviours seem devised to maximise conformity, minimising individual differences; thus a six-year-old 'doesn't like to be different from the other children in

* Differences between groups were assessed using the t test.

[1] $t = 3·06$, df = 55, $p < 0·01$.

[2] $t = 4·07$, df = 24, $p < 0·001$.

the way she dresses. She likes to be the same as the other children. She once had a schoolbag that was not like the rest of them, not on her back, and she felt ashamed.' At other times, the child, through his fastidiousness, endeavours to outshine his peers. Occasionally, such concern amounted to a precocious fashion consciousness; thus a five-year-old 'likes nice things. She likes everything to be very neat. She likes her shoes with bows, and she's even interested in grown-up clothes and looks in the shop windows and says, "When I'm a big girl will you buy me a nice frock like that?" She likes people in their teens and early twenties. She's fascinated by how they look and keep themselves.' Parents frequently reinforced this defence by buying their sick child especially good clothes. This afforded them obvious satisfaction; for example, the mother of a six-year-old boy, speaking of his teacher, said: 'She always admires him, tells him how nice he is. Some children are shabby, but he's the nicest dressed in the class.' Through such indulgences, some parents clearly endeavoured to expiate their own guilt concerning the illness. As one mother confided: 'You never know how long you'll have her—so you might as well make the best of it whilst they're there.'

Another compensatory device for feared physical inadequacy seemed to be a tendency to increased talkativeness. As mentioned previously, a substantial proportion of the school-age children were markedly good on the vocabulary items of the IQ scale, and many parents commented on the sick child's constant chatter. One father of a seven-year-old said: 'She's like an old lady—natter, natter, natter.' Another said: 'She never stops talking—but if she does get quiet we know something's wrong—we ask her but she won't say.' Talkativeness helped to keep unpleasant thoughts and fears at bay and also arrested attention, thereby preventing loneliness. Some more perceptive children recognised this; for example, one six-year-old girl of superior intelligence confided that if she could be someone else she would be 'an understandable person who would be nice to people so that they wouldn't say, "You cheeky brat—I don't like you."' She was obviously thinking of her peers in this respect, for she added: 'They play with me for a while and then they get attracted to someone else—then I get lonely.'

Perhaps for similar reasons many sick children exhibited a heightened sensitivity and empathy to the feelings of others. Mothers of school-age children frequently told me how considerate their sick child was when they themselves were ill, tired or generally distressed.

The mother of a six-year-old best summarised this by saying: 'Sometimes I feel she's my mother and she's mothering me. Most of all, I find with her, if you have any grief she senses it.' Such empathy might also originate from the parents' obvious concern for the child. Many children spoke most warmly of the goodness of their parents, especially when they were ill; for example, a nine-year-old commented of his mother: 'She just does everything for you. If you were in trouble she'd do anything for you. She's an awful good woman.' In this context, one must remember that illness, even though it puts strain on the family, provides opportunities for very real interdependence, which, when taken, can have a very positive effect on family unity.

Coming to terms with the illness—the sick child's adaptation to his physical state

Finally, lest I paint too gloomy a picture of the stresses imposed by a chronic disease, may I emphasise that despite all the stresses and handicaps imposed by cf, most children cope remarkably well. Only two children out of the thirty school-age children flatly refused to go to school, and one of these was ultimately coaxed back and was attending regularly at the time of the study. Only three school-age children were sufficiently behaviourally disturbed to merit the label 'maladjusted', and only two children out of the entire group were thought by their parents not to have come to terms with the disease. The majority of sick children tried hard to please both their parents and teachers and did not make undue fuss concerning their symptoms. Some children showed evidence of a sustaining sense of humour; for example, one five-year-old called the smell she made in the toilet her 'secret weapon'. Other children had developed a sense of perspective such that they could see their problems in relation to those of other more handicapped children; for example, one six-year-old complained to me that the other children in her class wouldn't play with her. Then she added: 'When I ask, the children turn their backs on me. I think it's because I don't look nice. They all call me names like "skinny". I don't care, even if I am thin. I'm luckier than other children—some are crippled. I'm stronger even though I am thin.' In developing such defences and in learning to control their understandable anxiety in the situation, good close communicative parental relationships were of immense value; for example, one of the most secure children I met asked her mother: 'Why did God make me like this?' only to be told: 'I don't know, but there are some children born blind and some without legs, and you can run and see and play with your dollies and you're luckier than they are.' This reassurance was accepted by the child and her mother later commented: 'Now she feels not so badly off.' Similarly, an eleven-year-old, who gave clear evidence of anxiety in his personality tests, nevertheless managed to exist cheerfully despite his handicap. His mother said: 'He seems just to have accepted it as I have. I'm not anxious about it and I haven't wanted him to worry about it. When he's asked things I've explained it without emotion and that's how he's accepted it.' This mother's own positive attitude to rearing a sick child was formed with reference to her knowledge of an asthmatic friend: 'She was really wrapped in cotton wool. I used to resent that terribly. So much of it was unnecessary. They even sent her to a private school. That got my back up.' Other close communicative relationships were also of value to sick children, and several parents spoke warmly of the kindness shown to them by caring personnel. Children who returned regularly to the same hospital ward for treatment, and who had mastered their hospital fears, were frequently thought to gain strength from the continuity of the staff and the fact that they themselves were remembered. Seeing and often helping other more handicapped children in hospital could also be of value.

Intelligence was also a help in coming to terms with the illness. The more able children were not only more socially competent, but also seemed to have their underlying apprehensions more in check. In terms of their social behaviour in the classroom, children with an IQ below 110 displayed twice as many symptoms of unsettled behaviour as children with a higher IQ.

In addition, many children displayed great personal courage in the situation. Some even inspired their parents to greater therapeutic efforts. As a result, for instance, the mother of a six-year-old said,

'I have seen that child and thought her lungs were bursting open and she never complains. She shows so much courage and she's so anxious to get ahead. She could use her handicap a bit to get off things but she's determined to live—that's the thing. Determined to fight this. She knows she's a bit different from others and she's determined to fight this.'

Some parents noticed a relationship between the child's own health and both his will to live and his ability to accept his handicap. Improvements in his physical state, due either to hospital or home-based therapy, were a boost to morale. Similarly, those children who were in good physical health, despite the disease, were better able to accept its presence. As the mother of a ten-year-old commented: 'The fact that he's so well helps. If he was ill a lot he probably wouldn't accept it so well.'

Many children mirrored their parents' religious beliefs, and either hoped for a cure or accepted the illness as part of God's plan for them. These beliefs gave them strength. So also did their own strong attachment to their parents. When considering a child's response to his illness it is therefore important to remember that while he is under strain so also is he offered a very real opportunity to test the strength of the relationships which sustain him. More than ever, the sick child can be certain that he is loved for what he is, be it weak, timid, or 'protesting against the unfairness of it all'. As a consequence, feelings of closeness may develop which enrich both the child and his parents. Indeed, many parents preferred their sick child to his well brothers and sisters, and they felt that they personally had learnt much about life through their experiences with him.

12

Brothers and sisters of a sick child

'He does stupid things to get attention. He maybe does something that you had told him not to do, just trying to attract attention. At times he feels it that his sister gets more attention, especially from me. You can sort of a way sense that he feels a bit put out. I talk to him, try to explain things to him—he's a pretty easy kid to talk to. One of those kids that likes you to soften him up. He's a softee.'

(A father, talking of his well son)

Very little is known about the ways in which a child's illness, and his parents' consequent preoccupation, affect the other well children in the family. Perhaps this lack in our knowledge reflects a basic lack of care for such children. Understandably, the attentions of medical and nursing personnel are focused on the physical needs of the sick child, and few are trained, or have sufficient time, to consider the emotional needs of well children whom they may never have met, and who therefore exist solely as shadowy figures in the sick child's background. Similarly, parents, coping with continued crises or the exigencies of treatment, may forget all their theories of child-rearing, and pivot their attentions on the ailing child to the detriment of his well brothers and sisters. As a consequence, feelings of jealousy, guilt and resentment, engendered in such children by obvious disparities in handling, may cause immediate and acute pain, and contribute to long-term personality defects.

Well children are strained in several ways by the sick child's illness. First, almost invariably, they suffer some neglect— emotional, physical or both. Prior to the sick child's diagnosis, parents are worried by ephemeral symptoms and preoccupied by their attempts to restore the child to health. At the time of diagnosis they are in a state of shock. Subsequently they become anxious for the sick child's safety and depressed. Often their health suffers and they have less energy available for coping with everyday problems. The treatment regime eats into leisure time, producing a consequent diminution in play and relaxation. The need to escort the sick child regularly to the outpatient clinic can strain the family budget, leaving less money available for treats and surprises. In addition, the hospitalisation of the sick child can remove the mother entirely from the home, or reduce her to such a state of anxiety that she is unable to follow even her usual routines. Many writers (Freud, 1969; Robertson, 1965) have emphasised the way in which parental preoccupations of any kind limit the mother's perception and ability to respond to the emotional needs of her other children. As a result, the whole course of the well child's development may be altered.

Children of all ages view parental preoccupation as a rejection of themselves, and such feelings become strengthened if the parents inadvertently scapegoat the well child, displacing onto him their feelings of anger, engendered by the illness (Bozemann *et al.*, 1955; Burton, 1971). Where this happens, parents may become correspondingly guilty, and question yet further their own child-rearing abilities. They may endeavour to make amends, and experience a sense of uncertainty in legitimately disciplining all their children (Lindsay and McCarthy, 1974). In addition, in an attempt to compensate for their own supposed inadequacy in child-rearing, they may extend their over-protective concern for the sick child to include his well brothers and sisters. If they are forced to deny, or find difficulty in speaking of, the illness such inconsistencies may emerge unbidden and unexplained.

As a result, many younger children become confused and end up becoming naughty and aggressive. Older children may become resentful and angry. Frightened of becoming ill themselves, they may taunt the sick child about his illness or develop psychosomatic symptoms in a bid for reassurance and the required attention. Binger *et al.* (1969) found such difficulties in one or more of the well siblings of half the leukaemic children whom he and his co-workers studied. Rosenstein (1970) noted behaviour disorders, resentment and depression amongst the well siblings of cystic children, and Blom (1958) even noted jealousy amongst the brothers and sisters of children hospitalised for tonsillectomy.

But it is not just parental preoccupation which disorientates well children. Problems can be produced by the dominating attitude of the sick child himself. All siblings have to share their parents' love and devotion and where this is equably divided, feelings of loyalty, companionship and togetherness may be engendered. Where, however, one child regularly demands that his needs be met at the expense of the others, natural feelings of rivalry, hatred and jealousy may ensue. If the sick child is the younger child, birth rivalries may re-activate. If he is the older child, his younger siblings may become openly jealous of his obvious privileges.

Where the family has already lost a child, the stresses may be even greater, the well child's anxiety and guilt concerning the dead child transferring to the presently sick one.

In order to evaluate the ways in which the presence of a chronically sick child in the home could affect the behaviour and attitudes of well children, questions were included relating to these topics in the three interview schedules which were used with study parents. Fifty of the 58 cf children had well siblings living at home with them. In all, there were 112 well brothers and sisters—76 older and 36 younger than the sick child.

Changes in the siblings' attitudes towards the sick child, due to the illness

Parents were first asked whether they felt that the attitudes of their other well children towards the child with cf had been influenced in any way by the illness. Forty-two per cent of the mothers immediately answered 'yes'. A further 35 per cent said 'no', but upon subsequent, more detailed questioning revealed that such a change in attitude had taken place, so that in only 23 per cent of families was there no obvious change in the well children's attitude towards the sick child.

By no means all these changes were adverse. Some mothers spoke warmly of the extra care, protection, and lowered aggression which their older children displayed towards the sick child; for example, one mother with five children found that the four older ones 'all seemed to be helping' the sick baby. She added: 'they never thought of themselves at all. Quite the other way round. Perhaps we got no jealousy because our children are big and had more sense. If they'd been smaller they might have resented it.' Her comments were reflected in the findings of this survey. Table 29 shows that whilst almost half the older siblings displayed positive, protective feelings towards the sick child, younger children tended to react less positively. Indeed, they occasionally experienced extreme jealousy. In this respect, much depended on the age of the younger sibling. Very young children often showed no apparent change in attitude (and, in fact, two-thirds of the 23 per cent of families who showed no change in sibling attitude were composed of one cf child and a much younger sibling). Obviously, in such cases, the child was either too young to notice disparities in handling, or, because he had no standard of comparison, viewed inequalities, where they existed, as quite normal.

Table 29 *Changes in the siblings' attitude towards the sick child according to their ordinal position within the family*

Change in attitude due to the illness	Older siblings (%)	Younger siblings (%)
Gives in more easily to sick child	43	12
Less aggressive than otherwise	46	12
Feels protective towards sick child	57	19
Feels responsible for sick child's wellbeing	43	12
Feels jealous of attention received by sick child	22	29
Feels worried about the illness	47	9
Talks to or taunts sick child about illness	8	12
No.	76	36

The sibling's sense of feeling 'left-out' or resentful

Mothers were asked whether they thought that their well children felt 'left-out' because the sick child needed extra attention. Similarly, fathers were asked whether they felt their older children resented all the extra time that both parents had to spend caring for the sick child.

Thirty-nine per cent of mothers, and 26 per cent of fathers said they felt their well children were 'left-out' or 'resentful'. As one mother expressed it: 'I think they must do. I think they must sense it, that when one is getting so much, they're not.' Parents cited occasions when resentment was especially obvious; for example, when the sick child was first diagnosed or later when he had to go into hospital. Feelings of jealousy were accentuated if the sick child was showered with presents or given special treats on return home. Occasionally, one well child was thought to feel more 'left out' than the others. Most parents tried to work round such feelings by making a compensatory fuss of the well child: 'I don't put it all onto the sick child. I share. I give them all the same.' 'You have to sort of suck round him, sit him on your knee and say he's a big boy.' 'When there is time I pet her and comfort her to make up.' 'He gets very cheeky to get attention. We try to talk to him or buy him something. His Daddy would bring him in something from work to make up.'

The older sibling's response to the sick child

The most significant change in attitude on the part of older siblings was in their acknowledgment of the sick child's need for protection. Over half of the older children were thought by their parents to feel protective towards the child because of his illness. Such protection showed itself in many ways; for example, one mother found that her eight-year-old well child guarded her two-year-old brother from accidents: 'If he climbs up, she gets excited. I have to turn all the stools upside down.' In other families, the older child's protectiveness showed itself in more extensive caring behaviour: 'She would take her more and nurse her more, help her sort of a way.' Occasionally, such caring seemed thrust upon the older child by an over-stressed mother, rather than adopted from choice; for example, one girl, who was born eighteen months before her sick brother, became a virtual slave to his incessant needs. The mother explained her position this way:

'When he was born he had to have day and night attention, and I had to do everything for him, day and night. I couldn't manage and I had to use her. I couldn't cope and I had no one else to turn to and I had to get her to help. She was running up and down stairs with nappies and she reared them all. She pushed the pram up and down the garden with the next baby whilst I gave the child his physiotherapy. She does it now without my asking. She's very protecting, but she's done too much for a child her age. Others were out playing and I wouldn't let her out to play. She used to get annoyed—others got out, but she didn't. Now if she has to do too much, she gets very pale and her eyes water, but she knows he needs it.'

In this respect, older children were clearly faced with a dilemma. Although they might resent all the attention which their younger sick sibling received, they were old enough to appreciate that it was essential. Most older siblings therefore protested very little when asked to help with therapeutic tasks; resistance occurred only when the child was asked to help with non-essential functions. For instance, one mother confided: 'I asked my older son to wash the sick boy's hair and he said, "No, but I'll teach him to wash his own."' Another mother commented: 'I used to bath my son like a baby but his brother and sister said we were ruining him.'

Many older children were thought to protect the sick child from the attacks of other children; for example: 'He won't let anyone else hit her,' and 'If anyone comes in, she says, "you shouldn't hit him."' This trend was particularly apparent outside the home, even children who were indifferent within becoming champions without. Forty-three per cent of older siblings were thought by their parents to give in more easily to the sick child, and 46 per cent were thought to be less aggressive because of the illness. Sometimes this was only a partial lessening in force: 'He would pull her hair, but not hit her or hurt her.' Occasionally it was a total restraint; for example, one eight-year-old was thought to 'let the sick child torment him, so much so he would sit and cry and do nothing'. His mother commented:

'Bobby [the cf child] was so protected that he knew when he was only three that he could make his brother cry, yet my older son wouldn't hit him. Until that time I was the only one who smacked Bobby, but when he was three he was doing so well our doctor said he could rough it, and I came back and said, "If you feel like hitting Bobby now, you can do it," whereas before I would have said, "If you feel like hitting Bobby, tell me." But my older son couldn't at first. Later, he really hauled

Bobby across the room. When I saw this I had to control myself not to go and hit the older boy.'

By becoming protective in their turn, older children were clearly mirroring their parents' concern for the sick child. Also, in some cases, it was more than probable that such restraint stemmed from guilt on the older child's part, either because he was well whilst his sibling was sick, or because he felt resentful concerning the attention his brother received. Carefully guarding the sick child against accidents or injuries might serve to disguise the older child's hostile, yet guilty, feelings. This is well illustrated by a mother's comments concerning her five-year-old well daughter: 'When the wee ones are sick she's sick and worried, and says she's sick and can't sleep because they're in hospital. She cried every Sunday when I went up to the hospital, because they weren't home. She would say "I didn't do it" and cry if either of them fell.' This little girl would seem both to mirror her parents' distress concerning her brother and sister's illness, and also to be endeavouring to attract attention to herself by simulating illness symptoms. In addition, she was clearly jealous whenever her parents visited the sick children in hospital, yet felt guilty if they met with any misfortune. Possibly, for complex reasons such as this, many older siblings were thought by their parents to actually feel responsible for the sick child's wellbeing. In all, 43 per cent of older children were thought to feel this way. Some manifested this sense of responsibility in active caring for the child; for example, in wheeling him out, checking he had all his outdoor clothes on, and giving him his treatment. Occasionally, assistance of this sort seemed to stem from genuinely compassionate feelings; for example, a fourteen-year-old, helping with her brother's physiotherapy 'had tears streaming down her face. She was so sad. It was a deep sadness, not self-pity.'

Feelings of responsibility and worry concerning the illness escalated when the sick child was unwell or hospitalised and almost half the older children were thought to 'cry easily and break down; cries behind your back'; for example, an eight-year-old 'was upset' when his younger sister was sick. His mother commented: 'I had to bring him up and let him see her. He would ask about her when he was home from school. If she was kept in hospital sometimes he would cry.'

In families where a previous child had died, such feelings of worry and responsibility were magnified. One mother, describing her ten-year-old, said, 'She gets upset and tearful. I wonder whether it's because she's afraid he will die.' An eight-year-old boy who had lost a younger sister two years previously was described by his mother as tending 'to cry at night' when his younger brother had to go into hospital. She added: 'He wanted to know where he was. He asked, "Is he going to come home again?" You see, he can remember his sister dying.' Sometimes, such concern prompted comradely gestures; for example, a twelve-year-old wrote to his hospitalised brother: 'Be brave. I hope you're not lonely, and I hope all goes well for you.'

Jealousy was rarely apparent in older children. When it did occur, it was normally occasioned by very obvious disparities in handling; for example, a six-year-old was jealous of the fuss his four-year-old brother received. His mother said: 'He likes to be in the picture too. He likes fuss over him.' One mother found that by taking tiny presents to her hospitalised child, she stirred up jealousy at home. She explained:

'I wouldn't have enough money for toys for them both and my daughter says, "He gets everything and I get nothing," and I say, "If you were in hospital you'd get it." I try not to make a big difference between them. She doesn't like to see people bringing things to him. We make no difference, but unfortunately the grandparents do.'

Perhaps overt jealousy is less apparent in older children because by comparison with younger children they are more in control of the expression of their emotions, and can hide negative feelings. Also, it is possible that their guilt, responsibility and worry concerning the sick child may limit open expression of less socially acceptable emotions.

The younger sibling's response to the sick child

Generally, younger siblings were thought by their parents to show very little real response to the sick child's illness. Indeed, as one mother expressed it: 'She doesn't really notice the illness, it's the extra attention she's worried about.' In contrast to older brothers and sisters, younger children rarely felt constrained to give in more easily or behave less aggressively to the sick child (Table 29, p. 192). Quite the contrary, most mothers found 'they won't give in to him.

They don't understand he has a complaint and they want to fight with him'. A few mothers noted, 'They're just equals. They fight it out as strong as one another.'

Jealousy was the most frequently encountered response in younger children, and 29 per cent displayed it; for example, one two-year-old refused to let her four-year-old cf sibling be nursed: 'She pushes her off my knee, and gets into hysterics.' Often younger children felt that their sick sibling was getting something special—which they were missing—when he received his medicine or treatment. They were therefore keen to establish parity; for instance, a two-year-old demanded physiotherapy. 'She says, "Do my coughies too, Mummy," and I have to do her some too.' A four-year-old simulated illness to attract attention. Her mother explained: 'She feels she is missing out on something, without tablets, so she puts on a toothache to get asprin.'

Occasionally, younger children were obviously afraid that they might also become ill, and indulged in defensive jeering; for example, a five-year-old who 'frequently runs a temperature with a sore throat, and loves the special attention which I give him when he's ill, used to tease his 7-year-old sister by saying, "You've got cf," to which she would reply, "So have you". He would then argue, "No, I haven't. It's you who has to go to hospital to see the doctor".' Another six-year-old was similarly teased by her younger brother: 'Anna Maria's got cystic fibrosis. Anna Maria's got cystic fibrosis.' to which the sick child tersely responded: 'I can't help it. I didn't bring myself into the world. You shut up about it.'

Occasionally, jealousies of this sort among younger siblings were not expressed directly against the sick child, but found form in rebellious or cheeky behaviour. One four-year-old was described as 'very cheeky—you feel you have no control over him.' Another boy of the same age had 'difficulty in doing things he's told to do. He resents what is said.' His mother added: 'Usually he gets beat. He shouldn't really, for his sick brother gets off with a lot he gets beat for. Now he objects to that. He doesn't like it. He says, "Maurice did so and so, and you didn't do anything to him."' This little boy's father described him as having temper tantrums, 'crying all the time for the slightest wee thing. He must get what he wants, he agitates, does something naughty. Even if I reprimand him, he'll do just the same thing again, no matter how much I warn him about it. We have been trying to give him more attention, but it still goes on.'

Feelings of jealousy emanating from a well sibling were rarely missed by a sick child; for example, a nine-year-old said of her well brother, 'He doesn't like me. I don't know why. He teases and hits me.' A ten-year-old disliked his older sister 'because she's not very good. If she plays with me, she might accidentally scrape me down the face.'

Perceptions of this sort did much to stimulate reciprocal jealousy and resentment on the part of the sick child. In addition, many sick children clearly regarded their mother as their own exclusive property and resented sharing her. Thus, even if they were not the target or sibling rivalries, they resented any contact between their beloved mother and their well brothers and sisters. A two-year-old was 'jealous if her brother sits on my knee', a six-year-old 'would be jealous if I make the others kiss me. He goes raging and sometimes I get one of them over by me for a laugh and he watches and is raging and comes over and gets in the middle.' One six-year-old was described as 'going mad' and 'tearing her sister's clothes apart' if she thought her mother was showing favouritism.

Fortunately, not all sibling relationships were so fractious. Some seemed very sustaining, a fact noted with relief by parents, and admitted openly by some sick children. For instance, one five-year-old, describing her well brother, said,

> 'He always bes at school and I don't. He gets sweets and I don't. He doesn't get no medicine, only magnesia. He lets me keep his cowboy suit and I put it on me. I put his trousers on me to keep my legs warm, and when I have no trousers I keep his on all night.'

Problem behaviours displayed by well siblings

Parents were asked whether they encountered any problems in the rearing of their well children. Thirty-seven per cent of mothers and 28 per cent of fathers experienced some difficulties (Table 30 gives details of the problem behaviours mentioned. Often, one child showed several types of difficulty.) The most common problem was rebelliousness. The father of a six-year-old who frequently begged to be given physiotherapy described his problem: 'He has a strong will. It seems he's pitting himself against me all the time, seeing how far he can go. It really is a permanent war of attrition. Sometimes I reason with him and sometimes I meet his implacable will with my will.' Another six-year-old boy believed his sick brother got more attention than he did. His father said: 'You have to watch him carefully. If you told him to do something he would ask his sick brother to help him, saying, "It isn't fair. Make him help me."' Similarly, a four-year-old was described as 'very dominant, far more

Table 30 *Problem behaviours displayed by well siblings of cf children, according to their parents (some children displayed more than one form of difficulty)*

	%
Rebellious	13
Jealous/resentful	11
Bed-wetting	9
School problems	7
Accident proneness	5
Roaming	3
Stammering	3
Overactive	3
Excessively demanding	3
Asthmatic	3
Nightmares	3
No.	102

of a problem than our sick child. You can't please him. He's very demanding and he won't do what he's told. You always have to be playing with him and doing things. You always have to try and do things with him. He girns if there's nothing to do.' Some parents felt obliged to give physiotherapy to their well child, this being the only palliative for such woes; for example, a three-year-old who was previously 'very agitated' became less problematic after his parents 'gave him physio—just a token pat'. His father added: 'He did go through a strange patch, even if we talked to him and read. What he needed was a bit of physio.'

From parents' comments concerning problem behaviour, it was interesting to observe that very few regarded the well child's jealousy as a real problem to them. Some undoubtedly expected it, and thought it natural in the circumstances, others saw it as more of the child's problem than their own. Other difficulties such as bed-wetting, laziness, and accident proneness were thought to be more essential causes for parental concern.

Explaining the illness to well brothers and sisters

It would seem reasonable to assume that jealousy would be mini-mised and co-operation potentiated in families where the well siblings had been given some information concerning the disease, and the real need on the parents' part to spend extra time in caring for the sick child. Mothers were therefore asked whether they had ever undertaken such explanations.

Sadly, and not unexpectedly in view of the general dearth of communication concerning the subject (see above, p. 128), 53 per cent of mothers denied discussing the illness with their well children. Some mothers rationalised this lack of communication by saying: 'It was never necessary, they're not really interested in the illness, only in the attention.' Other mothers said their well children were 'too young to understand' or it was 'none of their concern'.

Where explanations had been given, they were usually of a very limited nature. Some gave a brief description of symptoms, stressing the need for greater overall care. 'I just said her lungs were not working properly and she needs a lot of care to be well, and medicines to keep her going.' 'I told them she had something similar to Peter, only not so severe, and she has to be kept warm and get more attention than the rest.' Others gave less complete explanations, contenting themselves with pointing out the sick child's greater vulnerability in play. For instance, the mother of a three-year-old 'explained about his tummy—not to bounce on it—for it gets very distended at times'.

Parental reticence in turn was mirrored by well siblings, and less than 10 per cent of them were thought to have talked about the illness to the sick child. Similarly, the majority of well children did not spontaneously mention the illness to their parents, or question them concerning it. Only 43 per cent of mothers and 27 per cent of fathers said they had ever been asked about cf by their well children and usually such questions dwelt more on medicaments than on symptoms of the disease. Even when queries were voiced some parents found it hard to answer. As one mother explained: 'I never give them a straight answer. I prefer not to answer at all.'

Evasive and inadequate communications of this sort did little to allay the anxieties and frustrations of well siblings, and may have contributed to the problem behaviours they displayed. It was obvious, therefore, that many parents needed help in deciding how best to answer their well children's questions, and how to give age-appropriate and anxiety-allaying explanations, where no spontaneous queries had occurred.

13

The loss of a child

'After he died it used to be I couldn't sleep at all at night. I got a lot of depression. There is never a day you wouldn't think about it even now, both the fact I lost him and that he suffered so much. He suffered an awful lot. Now I look at it I'm glad he did die. I'm thankful he was took—how would he have done if he'd grown up a bit?'

(*Mother*)

The death of a child is one of the most shattering blows sustained by a parent. The ensuing sense of guilt and inadequacy, the resulting loss of hopes and dreams, and the profound sense of deprivation compound to produce physical and emotional disturbances often of considerable magnitude. Inevitably, bereaved parents change in their approach to life, in their ability to work, and in their relationship to one another. All these problems are accentuated where the child died of an inherited disease, and where the parents not only feel directly responsible, but also fear further loss—either the death of another child already born to them with the disease, or of a child as yet unborn, who might none the less inherit the disease.

In addition, within our community, many mourning parents suffer from a sense of isolation. Whilst previous generations were assailed by constant childhood scourges, and were prepared for the loss of at least one child during his early years, infant and child mortality is rare today. Now, not only are parents ill-prepared to lose their children but they are also inexperienced in supporting and consoling one another following such loss. Traditional sources of support, such as the orthodox religions, have declined in value, and, in an increasingly long-lived society, the ceremonial aspects of death are becoming obsolete. Today, death has replaced sex as a taboo subject (Yudkin, 1967) and when the event occurs it is invariably passed over as quickly and furtively as possible. In effect, therefore, our community deprives many bereaved parents of the opportunity for openly expressing, and ultimately living through, their grief.

But suffering is not confined solely to parents. Brothers and sisters, if old enough, may also grieve, and fear for their own mortality. They too may feel isolated by the uniqueness of their experience. As Mitchell (1973) has emphasised, the child bereaved, even of a grandparent, is now a rarity in our community. Consequently, the loss of a sibling assumes even greater significance. Where children know the illness is inherited, and where they also suffer from the disease, their fears are correspondingly increased.

Of the 53 cf families I visited, 12 had sustained the loss of one previous child, 9 of two children, and 3 had lost three or more children. In all, 39 children had died out of a total of 209. The majority of these children were diagnosed as having cf.[1]

It was both surprising and saddening to discover the extent of bereavement amongst study families. Certainly, when planning the investigation, I was quite unaware that child mortality would figure so largely in the lives of the families I was proposing to visit. Consequently, when devising the original questionnaires, few questions were included relating directly to bereavement topics.

None the less, the majority of bereaved parents, most especially the mothers, spontaneously brought their loss into the conversation, and, without any prompting from me, constantly referred back to the dead child and the impact of his death upon the family. Talking of their loss appeared to afford such parents considerable relief; for instance, one mother commented: 'I find it a great thing to be able to talk over these problems. Your coming is a great thing. I've never been able to talk it over properly with anyone before.' Such

---

[1] This represents a total mortality rate of 18 per cent. Most of these deaths occurred in infancy. This is substantially greater than a similar cf population studied in the east of Scotland (Burton *et al.*, 1972), and far in excess of that expected in the normal population; for example in the United Kingdom the average mortality rate for infants born between 1966-70 was 1·84 (The Registrar General's Statistical Review of England and Wales for the year 1970).

comments not only argue for the therapeutic value of a study such as this, but also reflect the dearth of emotional support provided for bereaved parents in our community. As one father tensely commented: 'After the death, no one came.'

The effect of child loss on parents

Much is already known about grief, and it is now accepted that mourning reactions follow an almost classic pattern. Initially, mourners seem stunned and unable to comprehend the meaning of their loss. They tend to deny that death has occurred and wait hopefully for the return of the loved one. Later, after adjusting intellectually to their bereavement, they begin to feel an overwhelming sense of desolation. Bodily disturbances, indicative of considerable emotion, occur, the most usual being sleep disturbance, feelings of weakness, loss of appetite, sighing, crying, depression and preoccupation with the dead. While overwhelming in the short term, these disturbances can last for years, being particularly distressing on anniversaries.

In all these respects, study parents were typical. Few parents appeared to have anticipated, and unconsciously prepared for, their loss. The child's death therefore came as a considerable shock to them, producing feelings of numbness and disorientation: 'After the last boy died, and after each one died, I used to go into a sort of fit. I knew what you were saying but I couldn't take it in. I couldn't breathe.' 'After the baby's death I didn't realise—until a couple of months after, I just went numb.'

Gradually, as the significance of their bereavement became apparent, parents were desolated: 'It affects me in every way. I have no heart to do anything unless I have to do it. No interest in anything, that's the way it left me. I'm on tranquillisers.' 'I cry for the least wee thing. It started after I lost the child. It comes for no apparent reason. I can't put it down to anything . . . many's the day I dread seeing the light, but you just have to get up and get on with it.'

Somatic disturbances were considerable: 'My nerves have been affected. It builds up and I have to have a good cry. I have sleep problems. I can't get to sleep. My mind is working all the time. I keep making tea all the time, especially if I'm here on my own. I feel hungry and I have to have something to eat.' 'I thought I would never get over it. It affected my health. I felt very doddery—staggered when I walked along.' 'The time after the baby died I couldn't sleep for six months. I couldn't get to sleep. When she died I woke at five every morning and couldn't go back to sleep.'

For some parents, grieving was made especially poignant by the fact that intermittently they denied the child's death and imagined he was still with them. They therefore experienced a series of losses. 'After they died you think you heard them crying and you put out your hand to rock the cot. It was awful heart-breaking. Maybe for six months after.'

Memories were especially sharp and hurtful on the children's birthdays, or at Christmas when the family would normally have been together. One mother, who had lost two children four years previous to our conversation, said: 'It's still there on my mind—even now. At Christmas and on their birthdays I remember them. It's heart-breaking. Never a day goes by that I don't think of them. Even now. But you have to accept it. You have to keep going for everyone's sake.' Another mother said, 'I'm through it now. My first baby was eight years yesterday. I remember birthdays. It's then I remember. I don't go to graves and I can't say when they died. I remember them living.'

Several factors seemed to help parents in accepting their loss. First, if the child was in great pain prior to his death, parents were better able to see the death as a merciful release. In this context, one mother commented: 'If she laughed, she laughed till she vomited. If she cried, she cried till she vomited. In a way I was glad to see her go.'

Where parents had a strong belief in an after-life, this also helped by enabling them to visualise the child enjoying some alternative to his earthly suffering; for instance, one mother who believed in Heaven, said: 'When she died, religion did help me a good bit. I felt she'd be happy where she was.'

Parents who were unable to assuage the child's suffering or care for him properly themselves adapted more easily to his death. Thus the mother of two cf children said: 'I think God was right to take my last baby for I don't know how I'd have managed two cystics. I wouldn't ever have said I didn't want her, but I don't know how I would have managed.'

The age of the child when he died also seemed to affect the extent and degree of parental grieving. As with the shock experienced by parents at diagnosis, the younger the child at the time of death, the more easily his parents appeared to accept the event. One mother, whose baby died following surgery for meconium ileus, said: 'I never thought he was mine. I only saw him for a couple of hours. It greatly helped, not being so attached.'

Another mother who lost her child at a year, following a considerable period of illness, said: 'I used to pray—if he's to go, take him when he's young. It's hard to part with them, but the older they get the closer you get and it's harder to part with them.' A father added: 'If they have to die I think they should die before they can talk—otherwise they're just a bother to themselves and the rest.'

The child's response to his illness, and most especially to his impending death, had a decided effect on his parents' subsequent mourning. Where he was afraid in either situation, they felt failures, and this added to their distress. By contrast, where they had been able to comfort him, and keep him from additional upset, they themselves felt comforted. 'The child herself helped. The love she had, the way she was brave. Marie was brave. When she was trying hard this helped me.'

One mother who kept constant vigil with her eight-year-old who died in hospital was obviously comforted by her own ability to keep the dying child free from fear. She said:

'She knew she was dying. She asked me all about dying that week. She said would she be put in a hole and I said, "No, only your body. The real you will be in Heaven." She believed everything I said, she thought I could make miracles. Even when she was really ill, she felt I would make her better. She was thinking of going to Butlin's and having a pretty frock and ballet shoes, and I said she would have them. But she kept smiling so much as if she knew and she was trying to comfort me. Then she said, "When am I going home? I'm better now," and sure enough she was. From being blue—her lips and her nails—she went pink. She looked all beautiful, her eyes shone and her cheeks shone. She went real peaceful. She just said, "I want to go to sleep as I do at home."'

This little girl had been seriously ill for a long time prior to her death, and she had been acutely self-conscious about her thin, stunted body. Her mother had long anticipated her death, and she was the only parent I met who showed evidence that anticipatory mourning (McCollum and Schwartz, forthcoming) had been completed before the child died. As she herself commented: 'Nature prepares you—you have that many nightmares for years before. You get used to it. When it happens, you're ready.'

Perhaps this mother was able to support her daughter so adequately during her terminal illness because so much anticipatory mourning had already taken place. She had long since faced her own fears, and, as a result, was better able to concentrate on the needs of the child. Parents who were less prepared often found their own grief overwhelming in the terminal stage and this distressed them both at the time and subsequently. For example, one mother, who had lost several children, fought very hard for her remaining son. When his illness became terminal, she couldn't believe it. Sitting beside his hospital bed, she lost all ability to play with him or speak to him and could only cry. Her tears disturbed the child, who finally asked her to go away. 'He said to go to sleep, he'd be all right. He said I only made him sad.' Very reluctantly this mother decided to go home and two hours later the child died. His father, who was with him, said his death was very peaceful, but his mother was unable to forgive herself, and kept repeating: 'I made him sad and I just wasn't there. I just wasn't there when he needed me.'

Occasionally their conduct during the child's life became a cause for regret, and parents blamed themselves for supposed misdemeanours or inadequacies. One mother, who felt she had often lost her temper when her children were small, commented: 'Had I known I would have had much more patience, but I didn't know. That upset me for a long time after. Had I known from birth, it wouldn't have affected me so bad.' Another mother added: 'Looking back, if I hadn't worried so much I would have enjoyed her more.' Such feelings not only contributed to a determination on many parents' part never to feel regret again—a sentiment which produced substantial changes in their child-rearing techniques—but also led to a corresponding idealisation of the dead child. Thus, the child who was taken from them became the embodiment of all good. By comparison with their living children, the dead child was often thought to possess a special knowledge or gift. As one father expressed it: 'She seemed to know everything. She was wise for all the age of her.' A mother said, 'I can't forget her even now. The rest of them even now they talk about her. She had so much to say. She knew that much more.' Conversations of this sort, recalling the child and his ways, were very consoling to parents, where they occurred; for instance, the mother of the eight-year-old who died so peacefully said, 'My other children think she will be an angel. They think that's great fun. They want to know if she has many toys up there and what she gets for dinner. They talk a lot about her. I like them talking about her. I don't encourage it, but when it happens it brings her a lot closer to me.' Perhaps by recalling their dead children in this way parents were able to reduce slightly their sense of loss, and for this reason alone our conversations seemed helpful to them.

Occasionally, preoccupation with a dead child can reach pathological proportions, parents being unable to grow beyond their loss, and manifesting their fixation in many ways, for example keeping the child's room and toys just as he left them years earlier. There was no evidence of such abnormal mourning amongst the parents I visited, perhaps because all of them had other living children, including the sick child, who needed their care. Certainly, the presence of other children in the home appeared to affect the extent of grieving and parents repeatedly emphasised the need for them to maintain control of their emotions and care for the rest of the family. In a few cases, however, the grief of one parent was sufficient to alarm the other parent, who feared that it might become pathological; for instance, one father became excessively distressed because he could not stop his wife crying six months after their son's death. If he consoled her the tears would abate, but when she was left on her own they flooded back. She frequently broke down after they made love, and he felt that she must need medical assistance. This she refused.

Often one partner became so afraid of reactivating sadness in the other that conversation concerning the dead child ceased; for instance, one man said: 'I could talk about anything but that. I keep on the bright side to keep my wife happy. I couldn't talk over the loss of the babies for fear of upsetting her.' Similarly, two wives commented:

'I keep a lot to myself, even from my husband. I hide an awful lot. I worry an awful lot, but my husband took the other child very hard, so I say nothing.'

'I would hide some things. When we lost our last wee girl I could have cried, but I wouldn't let people see it. My husband showed it on him. He has carried two coffins out, and he got very depressed. I had an awful time with him. It got down under him. He went to work and sat thinking of the baby he had buried. He really was depressed. Now whatever I feel, I cover it up. I think to myself if he's going to get that down again, it's not helping me as well.'

Where one partner was very restrained, the other often found it more difficult to express and live through his emotions. This not only delayed the completion of grief work—that is, the breaking away from emotional bondage to the bereaved—but also created additional and unnecessary tensions between spouses. By contrast, those partners who were able to share their sorrow fully, often spoke of an improvement in their relationship. In this way, child loss often appeared to accentuate the tone of the parents' previous marital relationship. Where this was viable, the partners increasingly drew together for consolation, thus adding to pre-existing feelings of closeness. A father described it this way: 'When Sally died we got very close together for a considerable time. We were sort of consoling each other. After all, we were the two people most concerned about it.' A mother said: 'Our feelings for each other were definitely better after we lost the baby. We only had each other for comfort. Just him helped—he was there. You depend on one another for consolation.' Where one partner appreciated that the other shared his feelings for the lost child, this greatly accentuated empathy and mutual compassion. Conversely, where feelings were thought to be discordant, marital strain was increased. One wife, who separated from her husband immediately after the child's death, said: 'Her death was the final crunch. He didn't understand and he didn't care. He'd no feelings. You always were on your own.' Another woman, whose husband was unable to accept their loss, said: 'It made us apart for when he lost them he was jealous-minded and said they weren't his, and he didn't care. It was very hurtful. It's a terrible thing to be married to a jealous-minded man.'

In his classic study of mourning, Lindemann (1944,54) commented on the changes in wider relationships which frequently follow bereavement: 'There is a disconcerting loss of warmth in relation to other people and a tendency to respond with irritability and anger—a wish not to be bothered with others.' This would seem to result not only from the immense drain produced by grief on the individual's emotional resources, but also from an unwillingness on the mourner's part to be distracted from grief work. All relationships were temporarily discarded, except for those, such as that with the spouse, which facilitated preoccupation with the deceased. As a result, some of the parents I spoke to even found themselves becoming irritable with their remaining children: 'With my other children I felt a blankness. They didn't seem to be mine at all. Time helped. It just got less and less.'

Occasionally, the child's death gave parents a sense of being fated, or singled out for punishment: 'It just seemed to be as if we weren't meant to have any children at all.' Naturally, these feelings were accentuated whenever parents had sustained the loss of more than one child. Consequent feelings of frustration produced hostility which was directed at the apparently uncaring wider world. One mother commented of this phase in her life: 'I had a grudge against people. I sort of felt why had it happened to me. I didn't like to see wee babies or watch them on TV.'

Often such hostility was vented against medical personnel, whose efforts had proved so ineffectual. This was especially true of fathers, some of whom were very bitter in their comments. For example, one said:

'I get the feeling that doctors are inadequate; for example, our son was not diagnosed as cf until after the autopsy. It was like putting a car into the garage and getting it back not working properly. Someone was not doing his job properly. I don't have the same faith in doctors as I used to. I think it's the hospital doctors I'm not too sure of. I wonder if they're fully qualified or experimenting at my expense. I'm disillusioned. I wish they'd learn somewhere else.'

Similarly, a mother commented:

'She died suddenly in bed. No one complained to their doctor as much as I did, yet she was never on treatment. Our doctor said I was making a fuss about nothing—he thought she'd taken whooping cough and bronchitis out of it, but I knew she was really sick and sore. But she went to bed this night and we got her dead next morning. It was an awful blow. I thought, can no doctor be trusted?'

Hostility towards medical personnel was rarely expressed openly, partly because most parents realised that this was of little advantage once the child was dead, and partly because, as one mother commented, 'you never can start an argument with them—for you never know the day when you might have to go back to them for something.'

Feelings engendered by loss were not comfortable feelings and many parents endeavoured to escape from them by increased activity. One typical father said: 'I find the best thing for me is to occupy myself with something—anything at all—something to take my mind off it, so that I can't brood on it.' Working, if it involved change and activity, was welcomed. Outside employment seemed especially desirable. Conversely, desk jobs seemed of little help. One father I spoke to found, 'At the time the boy died, I couldn't stand being in, so I decided to quit the business and go into farming again.' Similarly, some mothers found that being at home increased their depression, and the only antidote was 'to get done up, to do my face up, and force myself to go somewhere with the children.'

Over-activity produced fatigue, which accentuated depression and anxiety. As a consequence, some parents found themselves losing their previous *joie de vivre* and becoming 'much more serious'. This was certainly accentuated where the exigencies of travelling considerable distances to and from the hospital during the terminal illness had left the parents in debt. As one father explained: 'When she was dying our car wasn't one hundred per cent and the fellows round here got fed up with us asking to borrow theirs. No one offered help, not even a social worker. We had to take taxis. In the end, we were left with a lot of debt.' During the child's last illness many parents were so emotionally involved that they unthinkingly sacrificed all they possessed to be constantly with the child. It was only later that they sadly counted the cost, at which time they were out of touch with the hospital social work department, and unable to receive material assistance.

Almost invariably the loss of a child throws in question all the assumptions upon which parents had previously based their lives. Instead of being rewarded for their care and concern, they are punished by their loss. Many therefore feel disorientated, as if the world had been set on its ear. Some wonder if there is any justice left. Frequently, they voice such feelings, and if they can be shown some reason for the tragedy this helps them to accept it. For example, a middle-aged mother who had lost her last born said: 'When the baby died, I wouldn't pray too much for I felt God was too hard. I told my daughter, but she said, "God's only trying you out to see if you can take it." Now if I'm down and out, I can pray and this gives me strength to go on.' Where a religious adviser was approached by a parent and found wanting in terms of the reason he advanced for the occurrence, great despair and disorientation was obvious; for instance, one father was told, 'Don't worry. He's in good hands now.' He bitterly observed: 'That's no answer to an adult person.'

Some mothers found it easier to accept their loss when they compared it with the possibility of losing their husbands. One confided: 'It once crossed my mind that as long as my husband was here all was well. If I'd heard he was going to die it would be a lot worse. I think it is the hardest thing if a father or mother is taken from a family. As long as my husband is here we can go on together and it's not too bad.' Another woman, whose husband had sustained a serious accident soon after they were married, said: 'I think God let my husband live and gave me these other crosses. If He had taken my husband it would have been worse. I'm thankful God left it the way He did.' Full acceptance of their loss seemed only possible where parents were able to perceive some meaning in the death, whether the meaning was in terms of preventing the child from suffering, giving the other children in the family a greater chance, or seeing it as a cross to be borne as an exercise in piety.

The response of parents to child loss due to an inherited disease
From the foregoing comments, it is obvious that any parent losing a child, from whatever cause, is subjected to considerable emotional and physical distress. But parents who already have another affected child, or who anticipate that any later-born child might also inherit the same disease, face additional problems. First, and common to both, is a feeling of hopelessness. As one father put it: 'The least little hope would make all the difference in the world—but we didn't even have that.' Parents cannot replan their future without taking account of the fact that they may be called upon to face the same difficulties and loss at a later date. They become acutely pessimistic, seeing only sadness as their lot. Faith in caring personnel is often weakened, and any sense of isolation accentuated. Parents feel that other people may empathise with one death, but not with a continuing saga—as one father observed: 'People don't want to hear repeated worries.' Often feelings of isolation were realistic. Where

parents attempted to explain to friends and neighbours that the child died of an inherited disease and some of their other children might also die, they were met with hostility. One mother said: 'The way they look at it round here, they think it's something terrible and infectious. They wouldn't let their children mix with my other children. They're deliberately kept away. . . . They always talk—they wonder there's nothing can be done.' Another mother said: 'My sister-in-law says, "It's awful to have these children—cruel to them." It upsets me for a while, it makes me very much on the defensive. People are very cruel.'

Hostile comments from family and friends added to the parents' own inherent sense of guilt, as one mother, who had lost a first-born son, said: 'I often wish he hadn't been born—for he didn't ask to be born, and if I'd known or thought we would pass on this disease, he'd never have been born.' One mother, who said she had not been told the disease was inherited until she had lost three children, commented: 'If I had known I wouldn't have had any more. It does make me feel guilty having so many. I think it's because they've suffered—they definitely must suffer having their lungs affected.' Where parents had knowingly conceived another affected child, guilt was even more marked; for instance, one father commented: 'I do feel very guilty. When we knew that the first one, who died, had it, really and truly we should never have had any more.'

Guilt and pessimism concerning the future contributed to a tendency to denial. Parents who had lost a child did not wish to think a later-born child might also have the disease, and even highly intelligent parents were averse to testing their other previously-born, apparently well children to see if they also had the disease. One such mother became markedly anxious when screening facilities were offered to her and said her husband would never allow it. She then consoled herself by thinking: 'I suppose it wouldn't matter, not having treatment, if they didn't have any signs of symptoms.' As mentioned above (see p. 24), the only mother who did not herself seek medical help for a later-born cf child had previously lost a child, and was defending herself from the possibility of repetition.

Once the implications of the genetic nature of the disease were fully understood, the majority of mothers who had lost previous children became terrified of conceiving again. As one mother said: 'I would feel very guilty having another now. I would dread the nine months, and dread the birth and being told he or she would have cf.'

Strain in marriage due to the loss of a child with an inherited disease

Understandably, fear of further conception contributed to a general sense of strain, most especially on the part of the mother. Significantly more mothers who had lost previous children with cf reported strain in their marriage when compared with cf mothers who had no experience of child loss.[1] Such feelings existed whatever the form of contraception used; for example, one mother who used the pill said: 'I would never think of intercourse now. My husband doesn't understand, but I'm afraid to conceive, so I don't have any intercourse. He gets very angry with me—he doesn't feel the same way as me.' Where personal or religious scruples prevented the use of adequate contraceptive devices, strain was maximised, and several Catholic mothers spoke of their difficulty in this respect.

'We don't want to have another child under any circumstances, but our religion doesn't allow contraception—so we have this big problem, which we haven't sorted out at all. I don't mind it so much, but he does, I know. It leads to discontent and edginess.'

'I'm frightened stiff of becoming pregnant now. I love babies, but I'm really frightened now of bringing one into the world, knowing what the result will be. It puts a great strain on our physical relationship. He notices it, but he doesn't get angry. He understands I'm frightened stiff of coming down. He'd like intercourse every few weeks but far less would do me now, though I know it's not right taking it out on him.'

Stress during subsequent pregnancies due to the loss of a child with an inherited disease

Where, inadvertently, further conception took place, mothers who had lost previous children reported significantly more emotional distress during pregnancy than mothers who had not lost children with cf.[2] As one mother described it: 'I was so worried in case I had another cystic baby, it got that I couldn't eat, and vomited every-

[1] Differences between the groups in this respect were assessed using the χ^2 test. $\chi^2 = 3\cdot84$, df = 1, p < 0·05.

[2] Differences between the reported emotional stress during pregnancy of mothers with no previous loss and mothers who had lost one child were analysed using the t test. t = 3·17, df = 44, p < 0·001. Differences between the reported emotional stress during pregnancy of mothers with no previous loss and mothers who had lost two children were analysed using the same test. t = 5·39, df = 41, p < 0·001.

thing I did eat.' Another mother added: 'I was inclined to cry far more. I just dreaded he was going to be born and then I'd be told about cf.'

Where the awaited baby was actually diagnosed as having the disease the parents' sense of anguish was considerable. The sense of shock sustained by parents at diagnosis has already been described above (see p. 39), and it is not proposed to reiterate earlier comments here. Suffice it to say that the distress of previously bereaved parents was maximal. As one mother explained: 'I just broke down. I thought of the other two. My GP put me on tranquillisers right away, but nothing helped. I'm still not adjusted to it. I just lie sleepless at night. I know he's got it. I know they're doing everything for him—but when you know all—it's desperately upsetting.' Many parents became utterly pessimistic; for example, a mother said: 'There's no future for this child, and it's going to come some day sooner or later, and you must just get that into your mind.' Then she added: 'I get into panics at times and feel like doing myself in.' A father added: 'As far as losing the child is concerned, you have to be realistic. It can happen. It's always there at the back of your mind.' Another father commented: 'I've never thought of my daughter growing up. I've never thought of her getting even to school age. I know it's possible but I always think there's a chance we can lose her. I can never convince myself she's going to live.'

The erosion of their previous faith in medical science contributed to the parents' feelings of pessimism. A mother, who opposed the hospitalisation of her second cf child, said: 'I feel there is nothing to gain. It would be the same as before—no new treatment. I just feel they don't know anything. They've done no good. More harm than good. My daughter, who died, hated the hospital and was frightened of it, and when I took her in they did no good. It was just torture for her.' A father commented of clinic visits: 'What's the point if they can't do anything?'

Often the parents' pessimism was echoed by caring staff and relatives; for example, one GP told a mother who had lost two previous children: 'You know what is ahead of you, if she's going to die you've got to be prepared for it.' Another GP was thought to say: 'Why prolong life? When she grows up she'll have an awful lot more problems.' A mother said her relatives 'thought it would be better if God was going to take him as a baby, and if he takes a turn, they say he won't do.'

Frequently, parents hoped that if the later-born cf child was to die, he would die speedily whilst still an infant, thereby lessening their anticipated anguish. One mother, who had threatened miscarriage during pregnancy, said: 'I feel it would have been better for us all and him if he had been allowed to continue as a miscarriage. I feel the threatened miscarriage should have been allowed to go on.' Remembering a previous son's pain, one father commented of his later-born cf child:

'When he was in hospital I prayed he'd be taken away. I didn't want him to come home and sit in a corner. . . . I felt if it was God's will he was taken away, it was better for him to go then. I couldn't bear him to mope away—not get out to play. I'd break my heart for him.'

Some parents admitted to deliberately endeavouring at the outset to diminish their emotional bond with this later-born sick child. When he was hospitalised, especially as an infant, they declined to visit; as one mother said: 'I would rather not see him at all. My husband went up and said it wouldn't be long before he died, and I preferred not to see him at all.' Another mother commented: 'I told my husband to go, for the child was very ill. I didn't go. I wanted to go, but I didn't want to go. I didn't want to see him suffering.'

If the ailing infant survived, there was often some ambivalence in the parents' initial attitude to him. Comments such as, 'If they can't be reasonably normal I feel they would be better dead,' were typical. However, as the child grew, it became increasingly difficult not to love him, and the parents' more positive attitudes strengthened: 'The longer he lives, the harder it would be to part with him. He's very affectionate and now I would spare no effort in order to keep him alive as long as possible.' None the less, worries concerning the child's survival persisted. Some of these related to his objective physical condition: 'He looked like a Biafran. I was dreadful afraid for to take him home. I nearly had a heart attack when I saw what he looked like.' Other fears related more closely to parental experiences with the now dead child: 'I had an awful fear whenever he came home. Every time he got ready for his bottle I was so afraid of him in case he wouldn't take it or would be sick—the way she was.' One father admitted to being afraid 'to be left on my own with the child' and argued with his wife whenever she wanted to go out and leave him to babysit. Similarly, relatives became less eager to lend a hand with the sick child; as one mother explained: 'They are afraid he is going to die overnight too—which he won't—but they are afraid. They'll look after our well boy—but not him.'

Change in child-rearing methods and parental expectations for the sick child

Most parents who had lost a previous child with cf found difficulty in maintaining optimism with the later-born cf child. A real sense of doom clouded their expectations. As one mother expressed it: 'On account of the other two dying I had it in my mind that he would be dead and all in a couple of weeks. I didn't know much about it. I thought they only lived that long.' A father said: 'I don't know how long he'll be here. You don't know if they'll do, do you?'

Every small setback or difficulty reactivated this basic fear of death. If the child had feeding problems: 'I felt she could die over that—not getting fed properly.' If the child caught a cold, some mothers became frantic: 'To me a cold is the beginning of a death. I know they can die with a cold. She's doing damage to her lungs the more colds she takes.' 'Sometimes I do get worried if she's not well. I lost my other child so quickly. She was alive one day and dead three days later. I get frightened if she has a cough now and think is this her last night?'

Understandably, parents tended to take especial care of this vulnerable child (Green and Solnit, 1964). Rooms were kept extra warm; children were prevented from playing out of doors. One mother of a seven-year-old girl, who had lost two previous children, never bathed the child upstairs, brought warm water to wash her in front of the fire, never let her outside without a scarf and coat, and regularly carried her to Sunday School class at the end of the street—all this despite the fact that the child enjoyed remarkably good health. This mother found herself repeatedly nagging the child: 'If you take a cold, you'll have to go to hospital.' She admitted: 'It hurts me after I've said it, but I don't seem able to control it. I worry a lot. I regret depriving her and being so fussy and worrying so much.'

As might be predicted from the early study of Green and Solnit (1964), this sad, over-protected, little girl displayed behavioural difficulties from earliest days. Her mother commented: 'She was a very yappy, worried baby, always crying. People used to say she was spoilt—but she wasn't. She was crying, yapping, winging about something—a child that just wasn't happy.'

As mentioned in chapter 10 (p. 153), parents who had lost children changed most in their rearing methods and expectations for the sick child, tending to overprotect.[1] Less was expected of the later-born cf child in all ways, and whatever misdemeanours he initiated he was speedily forgiven: 'Whatever he does he gets off with it.' Parents justified overprotection in terms of the child, saying it was only right to give him as happy a time as possible, for 'you never know how long you'll have them'. Similarly, parents admitted to overprotecting this child in order to avoid additional regrets in the event of his death.

Parental inability to speak of the illness with the sick child, accentuated by experience of child loss

It has already been emphasised (p. 132) that many parents encounter difficulties in speaking to their sick child about his illness. These difficulties in communication were significantly increased where parents had already experienced the loss of a child.[2] Such reticence is perfectly understandable in view of the tendency on the part of such parents to view the illness as a death sentence; for instance, one father, asked whether he would find it easy or difficult to explain the facts of cf to his child, said: 'I think I'd find it rather difficult, like breaking the news of a death sentence to someone.' Another father commented: 'It is not right to explain to him—it is better not to tell him. I just see myself giving him his medicine, but it's not right to say too much.'

Even where the child was old enough to question the parent directly about the illness, or was obviously seeking information concerning the death of a previous sibling, parents felt compelled to evade the issue; for example, the mother of a ten-year-old said: 'He doesn't even know wee James died of it. When the consultant was here recently he asked, "Is there anyone else in the family who has

[1] Differences in the change in expectation scores of parents with no previous loss were compared with those obtained by parents with one previous loss, using a t test. $t = 2.22$, $df = 31$, $p < 0.05$.

[2] Differences in the level of parent-child communication regarding the illness, between parents with no experience of previous loss and parents who had lost a previous child were analysed using a t test. $t = 2.63$, $df = 36$, $p < 0.02$.

it?'' and of course Billy heard and wanted to know if wee James had had it. But I said, "No, wee James died of a tumour on the brain." If Billy did know his brother died of it, it would worry him. I know.' The parents' anxiety to avoid discussing the illness was reflected in the sick child's own inability to speak of it—a factor to be considered later in this chapter.

The response of well brothers and sisters to the death of a sibling

Very little is yet known concerning the effect of the death of a sibling on a well brother and sister. As Mitchell (1973) has emphasised, the way in which an individual child reacts will be governed by many variables, some almost too obvious to mention; for example, the age of the child at the time of loss, the degree of contact he had with his sibling, the presence or absence of immediate substitutes, the degree of his own personal stability and his previous experiences of loss. Perhaps for this reason, Rogers (1966) suggested that no syndrome could be identified specific only to reaction to sibling loss. Rather, as Binger *et al.* (1969) found in relation to leukaemia, considerable individual differences exist in the way in which well brothers and sisters respond to their sibling's death. Some children cried and verbalised their grief directly. Others worked it out through play activities. Some seemed initially unconcerned, yet over-reacted to a subsequent loss—for example, that of a pet. Others showed behavioural changes, but said little. Still others feared that they also would die of the disease. Rosenblatt (1969) described such a case, in which a six-year-old boy feared that he would die just as his two-year-old sister had done.

Where the dead child occupied a paramount place in the family, feelings of jealousy and rivalry during his life-time might give way to a sense of relief at his death. Such feelings, if recognised, could produce additional guilt for the well child. Cain *et al.* (1964) described a group of children bereaved of a sibling who became sufficiently disturbed to warrant psychiatric attention. In about half the cases, guilt was present, and, in some, still active five years or more after the event. These children were depressed and anxious, often feeling responsible for the death or believing that they should have died instead. Some had decidedly suicidal thoughts and evinced a wish to join the dead sibling. They progressed badly at school, and often showed evidence of accident proneness.

Obviously, in all these respects, the response of well brothers and sisters to sibling death must depend to a large extent on the way in which the parents respond. Earlier I emphasised (p. 190) that parental preoccupation of any sort can have a damaging effect on the emotional wellbeing of children, especially very young children who do not fully understand it. In addition, as a result of their loss, parents may begin to over-protect their well children, in case their lives also are endangered. Various studies (MacCarthy, 1969; Cain and Cain, 1964) exist, suggesting an impaired parent-child relationship following the death of a sibling. Such disturbances may contribute to psychiatric referrals during childhood and even later in adult life (Mitchell, 1973; Hilgard, 1969; Pollock, 1962; and Brown, 1968).

This study was not devised to elicit information concerning these topics; none the less, some parents spontaneously alluded to them in the course of our conversations. From the parents' standpoint, one of the most distressing problems was the initial problem of informing well children of the death. One mother explained:

'My two boys took the death of the first baby worst. I can remember their sitting crying. When the next one was born, and I found out he was ailing, I was worried for the children back home and how would I tell them. They were delighted to have another baby and how could I tell them he wouldn't live.'

Some parents 'solved' this problem by stressing that the dead child would continue to live in another world. As one mother described it: 'I told the others she had gone to Heaven. I never put it the cold way that she was dead. It seemed a nicer, kinder way to tell them.' Another mother said:

'My children asked a lot of questions about the child who died because they knew he was ill and the doctor came a lot—and the cot was all covered in. When he died, they asked where he was and I said, "God took him to Heaven," and then they asked, "How did he get down there? Is Heaven full of toys?" I found it very hard to explain to wee ones.'

Whilst stories about Heaven often prompted conversations concerning the dead sibling's activities in another sphere—which were consoling to children and parents alike—some especially sensitive children showed evidence of considerable fear; for example, one nine-year-old was described as becoming increasingly apprehensive.

'If she gets sick, she says, "Mummy, will I die? Will I go to Heaven like Pat?" She really is very sensitive, even now [three years later] she would cry and weep. The others are not so affected. She weeps if you say Pat is away to Heaven. She knows she's dead. Last year, when she went into hospital for her tonsils out, she fretted and cried desperately.'

This point was emphasised by a number of parents—the siblings of children who had died in hospital were often very afraid of hospitals and hospital doctors later. One six-year-old boy 'was afraid, for he was with us when we took her into hospital and she didn't come out. He thought hospital had sent her to Heaven and he kept asking, "Did she want to go?"' Such fear was also demonstrated when another sick sibling had to go in for treatment. As one mother explained: 'He always asks, "Is he going to come out again?"' She explained: 'You see he can remember my other wee girl going in. She only died two years ago.'

Children who were old enough to remember the previous child's death were usually more considerate of the remaining sick child, though this might be due as much to their greater age as to their recollections. Similarly, older children were often able to comfort their parents, providing both emotional support and a sense of perspective. One mother said: 'When she died I cried, but the other children said, "Sure, Mam, we all have to go—she's just a wee bit earlier than the rest."'

The response of sick children to the death of a sibling

Very little has been written concerning the reactions of sick children to the death of a sibling with the same disease. A lot must depend on the age of the sick child, though Lindsay and MacCarthy (1974) suggest that even quite young children are quick to notice similarities between themselves and the child who died. Even if reassurances concerning their health are given, such children regard them with cynicism. Parents in this study were not directly questioned concerning this topic, but I formed the impression that any negative reactions on the sick child's part to sibling bereavement were hastily denied; for instance, one mother assured me that her eight-year-old 'never associated' the illness of the dead child 'with his own'. She added: 'He's never thought that, but he does ask where she is. He says, "We'll pray to God and ask for our Marianne back." ' In this respect, the sick children clearly accorded with their parents' unspoken desire that illness topics should be avoided. Just as parents of dead children were significantly less able to talk over the illness with later-born sick children (as compared with similar parents who had not sustained such loss), so sick children from such families were significantly less able to talk normally of their illness when compared with sick children from families with no loss.[1]

One can only conclude that the 'wall of silence' (Turk, 1964), so often used in families of sick children to batten in uncomfortable feelings, is constructed with even greater strength in the families of the bereaved. Yet the need remains for all family members to talk through and come to terms with their fears and grief. The supportive intervention of a properly trained and helpful third party may thus be of considerable value to the mental health of all such family members.

---

[1] Differences in the degrees of ability displayed by sick children in talking over their illness were compared using a t test. Children from families with no previous child loss were significantly better able to talk of their illness than children from families sustaining such loss. $t = 2\cdot21$, $df = 44$, $p < 0\cdot05$.

14

Learning to live with a chronic disease

'I think the truth about this illness takes a long time to sink in, and when it does sink in, either you go mad or you accept it, one or the other.'

(*Father of a six-year-old*)

In the foregoing chapters I have endeavoured to pinpoint some of the stresses which arose for the family faced with the task of caring for a chronically sick child. Practical difficulties were legion, and parents were forced to assume extra responsibilities and cope with complex behavioural and social problems at each stage in the child's development.

Understandably, stresses of this magnitude were not encountered without upset and anguish, and as a consequence 36 per cent of mothers and 45 per cent of fathers admitted to feelings of resentment and bitterness concerning the illness. Failure to produce a normal child, feelings of being picked upon or singled out by fate, the social restraints imposed by the need constantly to give priority to the sick child's needs, all contributed to such feelings. In addition, as with parents of other chronically sick children (Easson, 1968; Bozemann *et al.,* 1955), many study parents felt a disquieting resentment building up against their sick child, who, despite their concern and often heroic attempts to give treatment, failed to thrive and thereby threatened to abandon them.

Such complex feelings puzzled and saddened many of the parents

I spoke to; for example, the mother of a four-year-old confided: 'When she is sick I get cross. I don't know why it is. I don't blame her—but I get cross with people. I can't understand it. If she is cross I get irritated with her. I don't want to be and I feel terrible if I am.'

Twenty-six per cent of mothers and 11 per cent of fathers felt isolated by the illness. Such parents complained they were not able to get out as much as they wished; for instance, the mother of a very handicapped six-year-old said:

'I hear of others going to dances and I think, "God, I'd love to go to a dance," but no one will mind your youngsters when you've a sick child. They're afraid. I do resent it in a way. I don't feel it towards him—not "if you weren't there I'd go out" —but I still want to go.'

Those few parents who hoped to lead a busy social life, travel, or emigrate, felt the restrictions most. One father expressed it thus:

'We've thought many times of emigrating, and we would have done it except for the illness—but not now. We'd love to get away out of this place—we hate it—but she's doing pretty well now and I would hate to take her to a climate that didn't agree with her.'

Feelings of isolation and alienation were heightened by the general ignorance concerning cf in the Northern Irish community. As mentioned in chapter 4, some parents felt they were fighting a lone battle in a non-comprehending world. One typical father commented: 'I always had questions I wanted to ask and no one to ask them of. He seemed to be a child in a million.' The mother of a four-year-old said: 'People don't really understand it. I think what annoys me at times is that they say, "maybe he'll grow out of it". I've got to the stage now where I don't bother answering them when they say that. I just let them say it.'

Mothers suffered from feelings of being over-burdened and unable to cope, and approximately one-third of them worried that the child's illness might prevent them from fulfilling adequately their responsibilities to the rest of their family. This was especially true for mothers with several children and such feelings were accentuated whenever the cf child required hospitalisation and the mother had to leave her other well children on their own at home.

Forty-four per cent of mothers and 49 per cent of fathers felt discouraged by the illness. Usually, such feelings predominated at times of maximum stress—when the child was unwell or resistive to treatment or when the parent himself felt ill or depressed. Others could unwittingly add to such feelings by being unduly pessimistic. In this respect, one mother complained: 'People would tend to discourage you, people who don't understand it—they take a hopeless attitude; for example, "Take her home, she's as well as she'll ever be."'

To combat such pessimism and to counteract their own feelings of resentment and depression, parents often deliberately cultivated more positive attitudes. Some sought to develop a sense of perspective by comparing their child with others, even more handicapped. Thus one mother commented:

'As you go on you just learn to accept it—you just say he could have been born blind or mentally defective. You compare him and you think "we're lucky". The only time you would worry is when you wonder how he feels. I don't know what to think about that at times. I've never given up. I'm a very determined person. I feel I've got to keep him going.'

Similarly, a father confided: 'At the beginning, I thought, "Why me? Why us?," but now I've learnt to live with it. If the child had been mentally affected it would have been much worse. Now I see that we are more fortunate, thank God.'

Realistically, some parents reminded themselves of the continuing improvements in medication and treatment, and the corresponding extension in life expectancy. Many pinned their hopes on a 'cure' and praised the research work sponsored by the CF Research Trust. Thus, one father said: 'The way I look at it is —if they say he's going to die I think he won't. They'll find a cure for it. I think where there's life, there's hope, so I'm looking forward.' Another added:

'I suppose though the disease is bad, there are worse diseases, it's not hopeless. Cf will be conquered like TB. If only we can keep her alive until it is conquered. I hope and pray there'll be a cure. Science is progressing at such a rate there will be something.'

Occasionally, the child's continuing progress was a source of rejoicing. The father of an eight-year-old said:

'The way she's doing at the moment I am very confident she'll become a woman. She seems to be doing exceptionally well, much better than other children, and now there's all this research going on. When we first heard about her the life expectancy was five years. I felt, "My goodness." I felt I had to make her happy for the few years she'd got, but now I can see a future for her.'

Positive, optimistic thoughts such as these did much to diminish feelings of self-pity and resentment but it could not remove them entirely. From time to time, unbidden, they emerged, causing pain and disquiet. To counteract such intrusions, many parents practised an instinctive form of thought blocking—either deliberately switching their thoughts to something more hopeful, counting their blessings, or getting out and about until they forgot. The mother of a three-year-old described it this way: 'I just sort of give myself a good shaking and say, "We are very lucky she is so well," and we go out to town for an hour or two. I wouldn't sit in and brood over it.' As mentioned in Chapter 8, many parents found work of great value in this respect; for example, one mother said: 'Since I had her, I've made a big effort to get a part-time job, and then when I'm worried I can get up and get out instead of sitting in and worrying all about it. I get up and go out and feel a lot better.'

Coming to terms with the illness

From these, and other similar remarks, it was apparent that most parents, though temporarily subjected to intense negative and conflictful emotions, none the less managed to transcend their distress and attain some measure of inner peace. As a result, only 11 per cent said they were quite unable to accept the fact that their child was chronically ill. The remaining 89 per cent felt that in some way they had come to terms with the illness.

In this respect, parents of cystic children closely resemble parents of other handicapped or chronically sick children studied previously (Henley and Albam, 1955; Chodoff *et al.,* 1964; Hewitt and Newson, 1970; Jabaley *et al.,* 1970). Despite all the personal distress attendant on their child's handicap, most parents function effectively, curbing their own more negative emotions, mobilising hope and maintaining a sense of personal worth. Feelings of resentment, depression, isolation and discouragement are rarely allowed to predominate. Rather the reverse. Where they exist, they are usually kept firmly in check—witness the mother of a seven-year-old who said:

'At the very beginning when she was lying suffering I was really discouraged and depressed. I blamed myself and my husband and I took it hard and had a chip on my shoulder and then later I buckled down and realised it was my child and there was no use harping on it. I had to keep her alive. I had to keep her going.'

Before such inner peace could be attained, it was essential for parents to make sense of the illness. Initially, most found their illness experiences at variance with their previously cherished beliefs; for example, the belief that punishment is not meted out haphazardly but has to be deserved, or the assumption that goodness will inevitably merit reward. Resembling nothing so much as divine retribution, the illness challenged these assumptions by appearing to punish unjustifiably, and negate previous good behaviour. In an attempt to resolve this discrepancy, many parents held protracted self-examinations, during which they assessed themselves—and each other—for evidence of guilt or sin sufficient to warrant such a reprisal. As one mother described it: 'I sat there crying, feeling "Why did this have to happen to me? I've never done anything bad."'

Inevitably, no sufficient objective reason could be found to explain the illness, and parents were forced either to accept it as a chance happening, or to evolve some other theory to explain its presence in the family. Unless such an ideological adjustment could be made, parents were seriously disquieted.

Because of existing beliefs, most parents found it too disorientating to view such a profound happening as a mere 'trick of fate', and most were therefore constrained to attach some special meaning to the event. Some saw it as an opportunity to improve themselves spiritually, and many of those with religious affiliations viewed it as part of God's plan for them: 'It's a burden you have to bear.' 'It's a chastening thing, sort of.' 'The way I look at it is God has just sent me a child to look after—maybe I got off life too easy and now here is a cross I have to bear.'

The parents' adaptation to the illness was greatly eased where they were able to see some positive reason for its occurrence. In this way, these parents resembled other adults facing up to life-shattering events; for example, the political prisoners incarcerated in Nazi concentration camps, studied by Bettelheim (1943). The morale of these prisoners remained good, despite acute deprivations, largely because they knew why they were imprisoned and could, in a way, see it as a compliment to themselves. The fact that the Gestapo bothered to imprison them meant that they must be important, and their political persuasions must be a challenge to the Nazi regime. By contrast, the non-political middle-class concentration camp prisoners could see no reason for their imprisonment. 'They found themselves utterly unable to comprehend what happened to them. . . . They had no consistent philosophy that would protect their integrity as human beings.' As a consequence, they were unable to cope with such a reversal of fortune. They deteriorated rapidly, anti-social and shiftless behaviour was common, and suicides occurred. More recently, Cohen and Taylor (1972), working with long-stay prisoners in a maximum security prison, witnessed the same phenomena. Whilst some men managed to adjust relatively satisfactorily to this overwhelming life stress, those 'with no workable sustaining ideology retreat or else fight in self-destructive ways'.

Taking each day as it comes

People who are heavily burdened cannot plan. The inevitable discrepancy between hopes and dreams and sad reality is too hurtful. In such circumstances, life is better lived simply, fatalistically, on a day-to-day basis. Such a passive life-style prevents the growth of unrealistic expectations which both contribute to ultimate disappointment and preclude the enjoyment of lesser things. By contrast, individuals who expect nothing and deliberately limit their aspirations both avert potential disappointment and, more importantly, are enabled to gain small happinesses in chance happenings. A classic example of this is contained in Solzhenitsyn's *One Day in the Life of Ivan Denisovich:*

'Shukhov went to sleep fully content. He'd had many strokes of luck that day: they hadn't put him in the cells; they hadn't sent the team to the settlement; he got a bowl of kasha at dinner; the team leader had fixed the rates well, he'd built a wall and enjoyed doing it; he'd smuggled that bit of hacksaw blade through; he'd earned something from Tsezar in the evening; he bought that tobacco. And he hadn't fallen ill. He'd got over it. A day without a dark cloud. Almost a happy day.'

Shukhov gained pleasure from what was because he prevented himself from imagining what might be. Similarly, 80 per cent of the mothers and 76 per cent of fathers I interviewed said they preferred not to plan or think of the future, but found the best way of living with the illness was to take each day as it came. Parents justified this philosophy in different ways. Some argued that cf children varied so much in their daily wellbeing that it was foolish to make any plans for the future. Others said that planning 'tempted fate'; for instance, the mother of an eight-year-old confided: 'We take each day as it comes, for I'm scared to think of her future.' She added: 'I don't want to think of it. I have this fear about her. When my husband talks of her getting married I feel, "Don't talk of that." It scares me, though I do want her to grow up and have a normal life.'

Occasionally, parents used the child's age as an excuse for limiting their aspirations: 'We just live from day to day and week to week. I don't think you really think much about a child's future when she's only four.' To some extent, this passive, fatalistic ideology may be reactive to the child's illness and used by parents as a defence against its potentially fatal nature. However, some parents admitted that they preferred to live this way, and would have done so whether or not they had a sick child to look after. As one father commented: 'There is nothing special about our approach to Sandra. We've never really planned for any of our girls. We just let life take care of things.'

In this context, it was interesting to find that few parents admitted to any extraordinary ambitions or clear-cut expectations regarding their own future life. Few had visualised their ideal marital relationship before the event, and, even where they had made plans, such dreams were very vague; for example, one father said: 'I never thought I'd get married until only a few months before. I never thought about it at all. In fact, I was in my mid-thirties before I did, and I never thought I would. I think you should be at home when you're married, particularly if you have a family.' Another commented: 'I didn't picture it at all. It's just one of those things that comes along.' Women generally had thought more about their future domestic life, but even their mental images were sketchy: 'I don't think I thought about it much. I was never too keen to go out a lot. I always thought of having four children—two boys and two girls—and now I have four, though not perhaps the way I'd hoped.' Another mother said she had planned 'Just to be at home with the children, just as I am, doing for them.'

Generally, parents' aims in life were equally modest. One mother aimed 'to have the family reared and each one in a fairly good position'. Another hoped 'to have a nice home, the way I would like things. I've always thought if I could have a nice home, I'd never be ashamed to bring anyone in.' A father aspired to 'get a good, decent job'. Another wanted to have 'enough material things to be comfortable and plenty of time to do what you want, to spend with the children if you want'. Basically, in terms of their aspirations, most parents exuded a gratifying aura of contentment; for instance, one mother commented: 'I am quite content with my life. I would like more clothes, more style, but nothing very much different. I've good friends and can get out and we have the kids and are very content together.' A typical father conceded: 'I'd love to win the pools and go on a tour of the world, all sorts of things like that—but I know what the odds are against those sorts of things happening, and honestly anything I've decided to do, or to get, I can get it.'

This lack of driving ambition, and this basic contentment with life greatly assisted parents in their overall adaptation to the illness. Table 31 shows that only a relatively small percentage of parents felt

Table 31 *Alteration in parental aims and expectations due to cf*

	Mothers (%)	Fathers (%)
Not attaining ideal marital relationship because of child's illness	16	28
Feels resentful of this	10	11
Not attaining ideal parental relationship because of child's illness	10	13
Feels resentful of this	6	0
Not accomplishing aims in life because of child's illness	12	2
No.	52	45

that their sick child's illness had prevented them from accomplishing either a viable marital relationship, a satisfying parental relationship or their basic aims in life. An even smaller percentage of parents admitted to consequent feelings of resentment because of supposed deprivations. Most accepted deprivations as inevitable.

Perhaps, in this respect, parents were assisted both by their own passive, accepting approach to life, and, as mentioned in chapter 8, by the fact that in the majority of cases the illness caused no overwhelming financial hardships. Whatever the reason, the parents' ability to live contentedly on a day-to-day basis, without excessive feelings of deprivation, was clearly of enormous importance in their adaptation to the disease. Had they been more highly motivated and aspiring, feelings of resentment and frustration would have been correspondingly increased.

The strength of family relationships in relation to adjustment to the illness

Several writers have already commented on the possibility of family relationships being strengthened as a result of facing up to cf together (McCollum and Gibson, 1971), and families coping with muscular dystrophy (Henley and Albam, 1955) and cerebral palsy (Hewitt and Newson, 1970) have displayed similar strength in the face of adversity. Despite all the inherent distress, 64 per cent of study mothers and 53 per cent of fathers still felt that their shared task had drawn them closer together. Twenty per cent of both sexes said their spouse had been of most help to them in coming to terms with the illness. Such parents said that only their spouse could really understand and care equally with them. Sometimes the practicality and the courage of the spouse was commented upon:

'My wife didn't let it get on top of her—so I didn't have to worry about her. She was able to cope so I could go to work knowing she would cope. That was the biggest thing. I knew she wouldn't go into a flipping panic if he was taken badly whilst I was away.'

Often the married partner helped by assisting in the search for meaning, offering some acceptable reason for the illness:

'My husband helped me greatly. I was sitting there crying and feeling "Why did this happen to me? I've never done anything bad," and he said, "You're being selfish. You're not thinking of the child. You'll give her a miserable feeling and that's not fair to her. It's your job to keep her happy. No one can guarantee how long anyone will live—I can't guarantee that she won't die in a car crash, so it's just not right to sit and brood," and now I realise how lucky I am to have her and if she did die at least she would have lived normally until she did.'

Parents adapted best to the illness where they mutually accepted responsibility for the treatment task. Women whose husbands helped at weekends or in the evenings, or who were at least shown some concern in their own right, adjusted best. Similarly, by actively caring for the child at some stage during the week, fathers were better able to accept the illness. A wife, who found her husband of immense value in helping her to adjust to cf, said: 'I think fathers have to do their bit. There is a burden there, and they have to realise it . . . in helping with the child they will come to terms with the illness.'

Similarly, parents were assisted in their overall adjustment to cf by the manifest concern shown to them by wider kin, friends, and caring personnel. Generally, family members were most valued for the practical help which they offered: 'I couldn't have battled through without our family. You wouldn't get the beat of them.' Close relatives were of less value, however, in terms of the emotional comfort they offered. Often this was due to the fact that they too were emotionally discomfited by the illness and displayed considerable tendencies to deny its severity; for example, one mother found her family 'no real help emotionally, because of their refusal to accept the problem. Both sides of the family tend to disbelieve the diagnosis and say, "He's a fine chap. He'll outgrow it." This gets us a bit exasperated. Now we take the view that if they want to believe that they may.' Another mother said:

'My mother is a very religious person, even to a fault, and when
I was worried about having another cystic child she said,
"Trust in God." She doesn't understand the depth of the
disease and I wouldn't tell her for fear of worrying her further.'

The desire not to hurt close relatives by stressing the severity of the disease was widespread amongst parents, and frequently this prevented true communication between parents and kin. This in turn precluded any possibility of mutual assistance in facing up to the illness: 'I don't tell my mother anything for I'm afraid of worrying her. She worries far more than I do.' 'My mother-in-law is too emotional. She starts to cry. There's no point in upsetting her. I can't tell her anything about the child.' Relatives and friends could only be of value as confidants if they were prepared to recognise the severity of the illness and accept the parents' consequent sorrow concerning it: 'I can talk to my sister if I'm depressed. I pack everything up and go round to her. It lifts me a bit.' In addition, it was vitally important that the listener should offer some semblance of hope to the grieving parent: 'I could talk to my mother, she would look on the bright side, but my sister-in-law wouldn't look on the bright side.'

Often, friends or caring personnel could be of more value as confidants than family members simply because they were not so emotionally involved. If the parent became depressed, they could better retain their objectivity and remind the parent of favourable aspects of the situation: 'My friends say he's doing great. They boost me up a bit.' One mother said of her doctor: 'She's the only person I know who can offer me a bit of hope. I go in feeling depressed and come out tons better.'

Many writers have stressed the way in which sick children draw closer to their parents, and in Chapter 11 I emphasised the fact that despite all the difficulties imposed by cf many parents preferred their sick child to his well siblings, and felt that their relationship with him had given additional meaning to their lives. Consequently, it was not surprising to find that some parents felt their own adaptation to the illness had been facilitated by the courage displayed by their children. As one mother said:

'I think she's helped me enormously—watching her. I've seen that child coughing and thought her lungs would burst open but she never complains, she shows so much courage and she's so anxious to get ahead. She could use her handicap to get off things—but she's determined to live, that's the thing— determined to forget this. She knows she's a bit different from the others and she's determined to fight it.'

Loving their children, seeing their courage, and realising how much poorer their lives would have been without them, many parents were supported in their struggle to live with the illness. Often their resultant acceptance of the sick child was very moving: 'He's never held me back in any way. Quite the contrary, he's been a blessing.' 'She's taught me so much.'

Religious beliefs as aid to adjustment

Seventy-two per cent of mothers and 40 per cent of fathers said that their religious beliefs had helped them to accept and cope with the illness. A few parents were even more positive saying that their religious beliefs had been of more value than anything else in terms of assisting them to accept the disease. Religious beliefs helped in several ways. First, by believing that the sick child was sent to them for some special divine purpose, parents were better able to accept the event. One such mother commented: 'A minister once asked me if I stopped to think if there was a God. I've never doubted it—I feel there's a meaning somewhere. There has to be.' Another mother, with two affected children, commented: 'I think God gives special help to mothers to help them. He's given them the problem and He sends them the help. These children are a message in this world—a gift. More than anything else I think spiritual help is more important than medical help.' A father commented: 'I think this is part of God's plan for me. . . . I think it is a slight task for I feel God will look after her Himself and I'm just there to help.' Such firm beliefs gave a meaning to the illness, which enabled parents to sustain all the disadvantages it entailed. Prayer and a belief in God's power also provided parents with 'something to rely on other than just medicine', which in turn gave comfort. As one father said: 'Doctors can do much with medicine but perhaps you can do more with faith.' In addition, many parents were sustained by the prayers and good wishes of the congregations to which they belonged. It was of immense comfort to them to know that others cared, and sharing their sorrows and their joys with the wider community prevented feelings of isolation. In this way, the closeness of the Northern Irish community greatly assisted parents in living with their child's disease.

Only nine parents felt that the diagnosis, and subsequent stresses, had challenged and ultimately weakened their religious beliefs. Two commented: 'I couldn't pray too much for I felt God was too hard.' 'I find myself continuously looking for proof that there is a God, some kind of miracle, any wee sign, but now I doubt it.' Such feelings were mercifully rare, and despite the many emotional and practical strains imposed on the parents in this study the majority were able to administer the treatment regularly, maintain a necessary aura of optimism and relate well to each other, their sick child, and his well brothers and sisters. As in some previous studies of parents of sick and handicapped children (Henley and Albam, 1955; Chodoff *et al.*, 1964; McCollum and Gibson, 1971), when reflecting on the family life of cf patients in this study I was left with the impression of family strength rather than weakness in the face of trouble. Indeed, many parents not only mastered the practicalities of their situation, but consequently appeared to grow as people. As a result of their own personal suffering, they felt themselves more able to empathise with family members and with others in the wider community. Many expressed sentiments comparable to those of the mother of a seven-year-old girl:

'If you go through life with everything plain sailing you're inclined to treat things lightly, but if you have a child like Sally, you're inclined to think more about everything. Her illness has helped me to understand other people's troubles and problems, and has helped me to face up to other problems more, and deepened my understanding.'

Some organisations which may be helpful to parents

Association for All Speech Impaired Children

Room 11
Nuffield Hearing and Speech Centre
Swinton Street
London WC1

This organisation provides an advisory service for parents and others working with children with severe disorders of speech and language.

Association for Special Education

19 Hamilton Road
Wallasey
Cheshire L45 9JE

Tel: 051-525 3451

This organisation exists to further the education and welfare of handicapped children, whatever the severity or type of disability.

Association for Spina Bifida and Hydrocephalus

30 Devonshire Street
London W1N 2EB

Tel: 01-486 6100
01-935 9060

This organisation aims to support children with either condition and their families in every way possible.

Asthma Research Council

12 Pembridge Square
London W2 4EH

Tel: 01-229 1149

The council aims at discovering the causes and cure of asthma and alleviating the misery and suffering from the disease.

Bath Association for the Study of Dyslexia

18 The Circus
Bath
Avon BA1 2ET

This association will advise on, or provide remedial treatment for, dyslexia.

Break (Holidays for handicapped or deprived children)

100 First Avenue
Bush Hill Park
Enfield
Middlesex

Tel: 01-366 0253

Break provides holidays for deprived, disturbed or maladjusted children, or for children with mental or physical handicaps. Brothers and sisters of children in need are also welcome, where it is desirable not to separate them.

The British Association of the Hard of Hearing

Briarfield
Syke Ings
Iver
Bucks

This association offers assistance with all problems arising from loss of hearing, total or partial.

British Council for Rehabilitation of the Disabled

Tavistock House (South)
Tavistock Square
London WC1H 9LB

Tel. 01-387 4037/8

The council assesses the needs of the disabled and develops a comprehensive rehabilitation service.

British Diabetic Association

3-6 Alfred Place
London WC1E 7EE

Tel: 01-636 7355

This association aims to help the diabetic to understand his condition and its treatment so that he can lead a full life.

British Heart Foundation

57 Gloucester Place
London W1H 4DH

Tel: 01-935 0185

This association sponsors research and provides information on heart diseases.

British Polio Fellowship

Bell Close
West End Road
Ruislip
Middlesex

Tel: Ruislip 71 75515

This association fosters fellowship between, and alleviates the loneliness of, poliomyelitis sufferers. It will find means of training members to be self-supporting, and it will bring those who need advice or assistance into contact with available sources of help.

British Red Cross Society

9 Grosvenor Crescent
London SW1X 7EJ

Tel: 01-235 5454

This organisation will help with transporting families to clinics, and can supplement the care of the sick at home, especially in emergencies.

Child Cancer Care

2 Annadale Avenue
Belfast BT7 3JH

Tel: Belfast 669748

A new organisation offering support for families coping with childhood malignancy.

The Coeliac Society of Great Britain and Northern Ireland

PO Box 181
London NW2 2QY

This organisation promotes the welfare of, and offers information to, any medically diagnosed coeliac.

Cystic Fibrosis Research Trust

5 Blyth Road
Bromley
Kent BR1 3RS

Tel: 01-464 7211

This organisation helps with, and advises parents about, the everyday problems of caring for children with cystic fibrosis. (Additional information relating to international cystic fibrosis associations is contained on page 247.)

Disabled Living Foundation

346 Kensington High Street
London W14 8NS

Tel: 01-602 2491

This foundation will offer information to the disabled concerning practical problems.

Family Planning Association

Margaret Pyke House
27-35 Mortimer Street
London W1A 4QW

Tel: 01-636 7866

This association helps people to plan their families and prevent unwanted pregnancies.

The Haemophilia Society

16 Trinity Street
London SE1 1DE

Tel: 01-407 1010

This organisation offers practical help and advice on all the problems encountered by the haemophiliac.

Handicapped Adventure Playground Association

2 Paultons Street
London SW3

This organisation runs adventure playgrounds for children with mental, physical and emotional handicaps.

Institute for the Study of Drug Dependence

Kingsbury House
3 Blackburn Road
London NW6 1XA

Tel: 01-328 5541/2

The institute will answer specific queries and provide information on drug dependence.

Invalid Children's Aid Association

126 Buckingham Palace Road
London SW1 W9SB

Tel: 01-730 9891

This association provides support and help of all kinds for families with a chronic sick or handicapped child. Help is given through counselling by trained social workers, a postal information service, special schools and centres for handicaps not otherwise catered for, and financial help in special cases.

Kids

17 Sedlescombe Road
London SW6 1RE

Tel: 01-381 0335

This organisation provides holidays for socially and physically handicapped children at a holiday centre, open throughout the year.

The Lady Hoare Trust for Thalidomide and Other Physically Disabled Children

78 Hamilton Terrace
London NW8

Tel: 01-289 0231

This organisation offers support and practical help to disabled children and their parents.

The Leukaemia Society

Hon. Sec.: Mrs Erica Dwek
28 Eastern Road
London N2

Tel: 01-883 4703

This organisation offers support and information to leukaemic patients and their parents.

Marie Curie Memorial Foundation

124 Sloane Street
London SW1X 9BP

Tel: 01-730 9157

This organisation offers advice and information concerning cancer, and provides practical nursing and welfare help in emergencies to families dealing with a malignant disease.

Malcolm Sargent Cancer Fund for Children

56 Redcliffe Square
London SW10
Tel: 01-799 6237
      01-373 5861

This organisation offers practical help to the families of children with cancer.

The Maternity and Infant Care Association

109 Leverstock Green Road
Hemel Hempstead
Herts HP3 8PR

Tel: 0442-3944

This organisation is concerned with maternity services and infant care, and advises parents about local services and amenities.

Mind, National Association for Mental Health

39 Queen Anne Street
London W1M 0AJ

Tel: 01-935 1272

This organisation runs playgroups, social clubs and special schools and hostels for young maladjusted and educationally subnormal boys and girls.

The Multiple Sclerosis Society

4 Tachbrook Street
London SW1V 1SJ

Tel: 01-834 8231/2/3

This society aims to help persons with the disease, both directly and by co-operating with welfare authorities.

Muscular Dystrophy Group of Great Britain

26 Borough High Street
London SE1 9QC

Tel: 01-407 5116

This group offers friendly help and welfare assistance to families coping with this disease.

National Addiction and Research Institute

533A Kings Road
London SW10

Tel: 01-352 1590 and 4517

This institute offers treatment and rehabilitation to those who have become addicted to drugs.

National Association for the Education of the Partially Sighted

Vincent Road
Highams Park
London E4

Tel: 01-527 8818

This association offers information concerning the education of the partially sighted. It also keeps an up-to-date list of schools and classes where education for the partially sighted is available.

National Association for the Welfare of Children in Hospital

Exton House
7 Exton Street
London SE1 8VE

Tel: 01-261 1738

This organisation is concerned with the wellbeing of children in hospital. It organises hospital play schemes and transport services, maintains an information service, and publishes leaflets, comics and painting books to help prepare children for hospital.

The National Council for Special Education

19 Hamilton Road
Wallasey
Cheshire L45 9JE

Tel: 051-525 3451

This council exists to further the education and welfare of handicapped children, whatever the severity or type of disability.

National Deaf Children's Society

31 Gloucester Place
London W1H 4EA

Tel: 01-486 3251/2

The society aims to benefit all deaf children through their home environment, their education, and the co-operation of the general public.

National Elfrida Rathbone Society

17 Victoria Park Square
London E2

Tel: 01-980 4204

This society aims at providing social facilities for educationally subnormal children and their families. Projects, organised locally, include youth clubs, holiday schemes, literacy projects, voluntary home visiting, pre-school playgroups and mothers' clubs.

The National Marriage Guidance Council

Herbert Gray College
Little Church Street
Rugby
Warwickshire

Tel: Rugby 0788-73241

This council offers private counselling for anyone who has difficulties or anxieties in their marriage or in other personal relationships.

The National Society for Autistic Children

1a Golders Green Road
London NW11

Tel: 01-458 4375

This society offers advice and encouragement to parents of autistic children. In addition, it arranges meetings between parents for the exchange of information, and it seeks to provide day and residential centres for the care and education of autistic children.

National Society for Cancer Relief

Michael Sobell House
30 Dorset Square
London NW1 6QL

Tel: 01-723 6277

This society aims to relieve distress, anxiety and fear among cancer patients and their families. It provides practical and financial assistance to meet needs such as visiting costs, convalescent holidays and additional domestic help.

National Society for Mentally Handicapped Children

Pembridge Hall
17 Pembridge Square
London W2 4EH

Tel: 01-636 2861

This organisation of parents of mentally handicapped children organises welfare, youth clubs, speech therapy, physiotherapy and residential centres for handicapped children.

National Society for the Prevention of Cruelty to Children

1 Riding House Street
London W1P 8AA

Tel: 01-580 8812

This society offers help to any parent with a problem concerning the welfare of their children or their family. The society works with families in their own homes.

Riding for the Disabled Association

National Equestrian Centre
Kenilworth
Warwickshire CV8 2LR

Tel: Coventry 0203-27192

This organisation aims to provide facilities for riding for all disabled people who may wish to do so, and who have been given medical approval. The organisation will help provide ponies for children whose normal range of movement is restricted to a wheelchair or crutches.

The Joseph Rowntree Memorial Trust

Beverley House
Shipton Road
York

Tel: York 29241

This organisation offers help to the families of handicapped children whose needs are not being met under the National Health Service.

Royal Association in Aid of the Deaf and Dumb

7 Armstrong Road
Acton
London W3 7SL

Tel: 01-743 6187/8

This organisation strives to help deaf people to help themselves, and provides trained staff, special churches and social clubs to help deaf people to achieve their full personal development.

The Royal National Institute for the Blind

224-8 Great Portland Street
London W1N 6AA

Tel: 01-387 5251

The institute cares for the welfare of blind of all ages. Recovery homes, Sunshine Homes, schools for blind children, and rehabilitation centres for the newly blind are all provided. In addition, it provides Braille and Moon books and periodicals and talking books.

Royal National Institute for the Deaf

105 Gower Street
London WC1E 6AH

Tel: 01-387 8033

This institute gives advice and information on all matters concerning deafness and hearing. It tests hearing aids free of charge, and runs, amongst other things, a school for maladjusted deaf children.

The Shaftesbury Society

112 Regency Street
London SW1P 4AX

Tel: 01-834 2656

This society provides special residential care and teaching for all physically disabled children, most especially those suffering from spina bifida or muscular dystrophy.

The Society of Compassionate Friends

Hon. Sec.: Mrs D. Bayford
8 Wentfield Road
Rugby CV22 6AS

Tel: Rugby 0788-5087

This society aims at comforting bereaved parents by providing the companionship of other bereaved parents.

The Spastics Society

12 Park Crescent
London W1N 4EQ

Tel: 01-636 5020

This society provides skilled assessment for spastic children, augmented by schools, residential and day care centres, hostels and training establishments for the welfare and education of spastics of all types and ages.

International cystic fibrosis associations

Argentina

Fundacion de Fibrosis Cistica Del Pancreas
Hospital de Ninos Republica Argentina, Buenos Aires
President: Mr Ignacio Kremenchuzsky

Australia

Australian Cystic Fibrosis Association
P.O. Box 229, Bankstown
New South Wales 2200, Australia
President: Prof. John Beveridge

Austria

Osterreichische Gesellschaft zur Bekampfung der
Zystischen Fibrose
Universitats-Kinderklinik Wien
1090—Wien IX, Spittalgasse 23
Attention: Dr M. Gotz

Belgium

Association Belge De Lutte Contre La Mucoviscidose
Ave. Plasky 186, 1040 Brussels, Belgium
President: Dr E. van Bogaert
Telephone: 36-76-44

Canada

Canadian Cystic Fibrosis Foundation
51 Eglinton Avenue East, Toronto 12, Ontario
Executive Director: Mr John Powell
Telephone: 416-485-9149

Czechoslovakia

Czechoslovakian Cystic Fibrosis Association
Institutum Evolutionis Infantum Investigandae
Praha 2, Sokolska 2
President: Prof. Dr Josef Houstek
Secretary: Dr V. Vavrova

Denmark

Landsforeningen til Bekaempelse af Cystisk Fibrose
Australiensvej 33, II, T.V.
2100 Copenhagen, Denmark
President: Mr Henry Jensen
Secretary: Mr Tom Jorgensen
Telephone: 07-29-34-23

Finland

Cystic Fibrosis Association of Finland
University Central Hospital, Stenbackinkatu 11, Helsinki 29
President: Prof. Jarmo K. Visakorpi

France

Association Française de Lutte Contre La Mucoviscidose
66 Boulevard Saint Michel
75 Paris 6e, France
Secretary: General Y. Le Vacon
Telephone: 326-69-04

German Democratic Republic

Arbeitsgruppe sur Bekampfung Der Mucoviscidose
Fetscherstrasse 74, 8019 Dresden
President: Prof. Dr G. O. Harnapp
Secretary: Dr B. Gottschalk

German Federal Republic

Deutsche Gesellschaft zur Bekampfung der Mucoviscidose
Loschgestrasse 15
D-852 Erlangen
Secretary: Prof. U. Stephan

Greece

Hellenic Cystic Fibrosis Group
Pediatric Department
St Sophia Children's Hospital
Athens University
Athens 608

Israel

Cystic Fibrosis Research Foundation of Israel
Hasharon Hospital, P.O. Box 121
Petach Tikva
President: Dr Ezra Elian

Italy

Associazione Italiana Per La Lotta Contro La Fibrosi Cistica
Roma Via. A. Fleming, 55 Rome
President: Conte Umberto Marzotto
Secretary: Mrs Ing Saxon-Mills
Telephone: 39-29-74 and 39-29-82

Netherlands

Nederlandse Cystic Fibrosis Stichting
Van Suttnerstraat 44, Gouda, Holland
Secretary: Mrs N. Huisman-van Rijsoort
Telephone: (01820) 16 109

New Zealand

Cystic Fibrosis Association of New Zealand
P.O. Box 241, Auckland, 1, New Zealand
President: Dr R. H. Caughey
Secretary: Peter C. T. Hayward

Poland

Polish Cystic Fibrosis Association
Polish Paediatric Society
National Research Institute for Mother and Child
Ul Kasprzaka 17, Warazawa
President: Prof. Dr K. Boskowa

Republic of Ireland

The Cystic Fibrosis Association of Ireland
21, Knocksinna Crescent, Foxrock
County Dublin
President: Prof. Colman Saunders
Secretary: Mrs Mary Carroll
Telephone: 895-005

Spain

Associocion Espanola Contra La Fibrosis Quistica
Avda. S. Antonio M. Claret 167
Barcelona 13, Espana
President: D Jeronimo Pujol
Secretary: M Pilar Fuster De Carulla

Sweden

Riksforeningen for Cistisk Fibros
Department of Pediatrics
Academic Hospital, S-750 14 Uppsala
President: Sigurd Dahlquist
Secretary: Dr Hans Kollberg
International Secretary: Mrs Cecilia Falkman

Bibliography

BARSCH, Ray (1968), *Parent of the Handicapped Child,* Charles Thomas, Illinois.

BATTEN, J. (1966), 'C.F. and the teenager', *Cystic Fibrosis News,* June.

BERGMANN, T. (1945), 'Observations of children's reactions to motor restraint', *Nervous Child,* vol. 4.

BERGMANN, T. (in collaboration with Freud, A.) (1965), *Children in Hospital,* International Universities Press, New York.

BETTELHEIM, B. (1943), 'Individual and mass behaviour in extreme situations', *Journal of Abnormal and Social Psychology,* vol. 38, pp. 417-52.

BEVERIDGE, J., and LYKKE, P. (1973), 'Psychosocial Stress due to Cystic Fibrosis', paper given to Australian Pediatric Association, Canberra, April.

BIERMAN, H. R. (1956), 'Parent participation program in pediatric oncology', *Journal of Chronic Diseases,* vol. 3, p. 632.

BINGER, C. M., ABLIN, A. R., FENERSTEIN, R. C., KUSHNER, J. H., MIKKELSENSO, ZOGER S. (1969), 'Childhood leukaemia—emotional impact on patient and family', *New England Journal of Medicine,* vol. 280(8).

BLOM, G. E. (1958), 'The reactions of hospitalized children to illness', *Pediatrics,* vol. 22, p. 590.

BOWLBY, J. (1971), *Attachment and Loss,* vol. 1. Pelican, Harmondsworth.

BOZEMANN, M. F., ORBACH, C. E., and SUTHERLAND, A. M. (1955), 'The adaptation of mothers to the threatened loss of their children through leukaemia', *Cancer,* vol. 8, pp. 1-19.

BRAIN, D. J., and MACLAY, I. (1968), 'Controlled study of mothers and children in hospital', *British Medical Journal,* 3 February, p. 278.

BROWN, F. (1968), 'Bereavement', in Gould, J. (ed.) *The Prevention of Damaging Stresses in Children,* Churchill, London, pp. 35-61.

BRUCH, H., and HEWLETT, I. (1947), 'Psychologic aspects of the medical management of diabetes in children', *Psychosomatic Medicine,* vol. 9, pp. 205-9.

BURTON, L. (1968), *Vulnerable Children,* Routledge & Kegan Paul, London.

BURTON, L. (1971), 'Cancer children', *New Society,* June, no. 455, pp. 1040-3.

BURTON, L. (1973a), 'Caring for children with cystic fibrosis', *Practitioner,* vol. 210, no. 1256, pp. 247-55, February.

BURTON, L. (1973b), 'Cystic fibrosis. A challenge to family strength', *Health Visitor,* vol. 46, p. 6, pp. 186-90. June.

BURTON, L., CULL, A., McCRAE, W. M., and DODGE, J. A. (1972), 'Some Psychosocial Stresses Related to the Genetics of Cystic Fibrosis', paper presented to third annual meeting of European Working Group for Cystic Fibrosis, Wiesbaden.

CAIN, A. C., and CAIN, B. S. (1964), 'On replacing a child', *Journal of the American Academy of Child Psychiatry*, vol. 3, pp. 443-56.

CAIN, A. C., FAST, I., and ERICKSON, M. E. (1964), 'Children's disturbed reactions to the death of a sibling', *American Journal of Orthopsychiatry*, vol. 34, pp. 741-52.

CALEF, V. (1959), 'Report on panel: psychological consequences of physical illness in childhood', *Journal of the American Psychoanalytic Association*, vol. VII.

CHODOFF, P. (1959), 'Adjustment to disability. Some observations on patients with multiple sclerosis', *Journal of Chronic Diseases*, vol. 9, p. 653.

CHODOFF, P., STANFORD, B., FRIEDMAN, B., and HAMBURG, D. A. (1964), 'Stress, defenses, and coping behavior: observations in parents of children with malignant disease', *American Journal of Psychiatry*, vol. 120, pp. 743-9.

COHEN, S., and TAYLOR, L. (1972), *Psychological Survival*, Penguin, Harmondsworth.

CRAIG, J., and McKAY, E. (1958), 'Working of a mother and baby unit', *British Medical Journal*, vol. I, p. 275.

CULL, A., BURTON, L., DODGE, J. A., and McCRAE, W. M. (1972), 'Some Aspects of the Influence of Cystic Fibrosis on the Development of Affected Children', paper presented at the C.F. Research Workers' Conference, Manchester.

CUMMINGS, S. T., BAYLEY, H. C., and RIE, H. E. (1966), 'Effects of the child's deficiency on the mother. A study of mothers of mentally retarded, chronically ill and neurotic children', *American Journal of Orthopsychiatry*, vol. 36, pp. 595-608.

DEBUSKEY, Matthew (ed.) (1970), *The Chronically Ill Child and his Family*. Charles Thomas, Springfield, Illinois.

DOBBS, R. H. (1970), 'Social aspects of cystic fibrosis', *Respiration*, 27 suppl, pp. 196-7.

DODGE, J. (1972), 'Psychosomatic aspects of infantile pyloric stenosis', *Journal of Psychosomatic Research*, vol. 16, pp. 1-5.

DUBO, S. (1950), 'Psychiatric study of children with pulmonary tuberculosis', *American Journal of Orthopsychiatry*, vol. 20, p. 520.

EASSON, W. M. (1968), 'Care of the young patient who is dying', *Journal of the American Medical Association*, July, vol. 295, no. 4, pp. 63-7.

EDELSTYN, G. A. (1974), Personal Communication.

EDWARDS, C. (1966), 'Cystic fibrosis and the medical social worker', *Cystic Fibrosis News*, November.

FREESTON, B. M. (1971), 'An enquiry into the effect of a spina bifida child upon family life', *Developmental Medicine and Child Neurology*, vol. 13, pp. 456-61.

FREUD, Anna (1952), 'The role of bodily illness in the mental life of children', *Psychoanalytic Studies of Children*, vol. 7, p. 69.

FREUD, Anna (1969), 'The Concept of the Rejecting Mother', in *Indications for Child Analysis and Other Papers*, Hogarth Press, London.

FRIEDMAN, S. B. (1967), 'Care of the family of the child with cancer', *Pediatrics*, vol. 40, no. 3, part 11, pp. 498f, September.

FRIEDMAN, S. B., CHODOFF, P., MASON, J. W., and HAMBURG, D. A. (1963), 'Behavioural observations on parents anticipating the death of a child', *Pediatrics*, pp. 610-25, October.

GIBBONS, P. (1974), 'Social Work Help for Children whose Life may be Shortened', in Burton, L. (ed.), *Care of the Child Facing Death,* Routledge & Kegan Paul, London.

GREEN, M. (1967a) 'Care of the dying child', *Pediatrics,* vol. 40, no. 3, part II, pp. 482-8, September.

GREEN, M. (1967b) 'Care of the child with a long-term life-threatening illness', *Pediatrics,* vol. 39, pp. 441-5, March.

GREEN, M., and SOLNIT, A. J. (1964), 'Reactions to the threatened loss of a child. A vulnerable child syndrome', *Pediatrics,* pp. 58-66, July.

HALLER, J. A. (1970), 'A Healthy Attitude Towards Chronic Illness', (in Debuskey, M. (ed.) 1970).

HENLEY, T. F., and ALBAM, B. (1955), 'A psychiatric study of muscular dystrophy. The role of the social worker', *American Journal of Physical Medicine,* vol. 34, pp. 258-64.

HEWITT, S., and NEWSON, J. E. (1970), *The Family and the Handicapped Child,* Allen & Unwin, London.

HILGARD, J. (1969), 'Depressive and psychotic states in anniversaries to sibling death in childhood', *Internal Psychiatry Clinics,* vol. 6, pp. 197-211.

HOGAN, R. A. (1970), 'Adolescent views of death', *Adolescence,* vol. 5:17, pp. 55-66.

HOWELL, D. A. (1963), 'A child dies', *Journal of Pediatric Surgery,* vol. 1, no. 1, pp. 2-7.

ILLINGWORTH, R. S., and HOLT, K. S. (1955), 'Children in hospital. Some observations on their reactions with special reference to daily visiting', *Lancet,* vol. 2, p. 1257.

JABALEY, M. E., HOOPES, J. E., KNORR, N. J., and MYER, E. (1970), 'The Burned Child', (in Debuskey, M. (ed.) 1970).

JACKSON, K., WINKLEY, R., FAUST, O. A., and CERMAK, E. G. (1952), 'Problem of emotional trauma in hospital treatment of children', *Journal of the American Medical Association,* vol. 149, p. 1536.

JACKSON, K., WINKLEY, R., FAUST, O. A., CERMAK, E. G., and BURTT, M. M. (1953), 'Behaviour changes indicating trauma in tonsillectomized children', *Pediatrics,* vol. 12, p. 23.

JESSNER, L., and KAPLAN, S. (1948), 'Observations on the Emotional Reaction of Children to Tonsillectomy and Adenoidectomy', In M. J. E. Senn (ed.), *Problems of Infancy and Childhood,* New York.

JORDAN, T. E. (1962), 'Research on the handicapped child and the family', *Merrill-Palmer Quarterly,* vol. 8, pp. 244f.

JOSSELYN, I. M., SIMON, A. J., and EELLS, Eleanor, (1955), 'Anxiety in children convalescing from rheumatic fever', *American Journal of Orthopsychiatry,* vol. 25, p. 109.

KNUDSON, A. G. Jnr, and NATTERSON, J. M. (1960), 'Participation of parents in the hospital care of fatally ill children', *Pediatrics,* vol. 26, p. 482.

KULCZYCKI, L. L. (1970), 'Adequate home care for patients with cystic fibrosis', *Clinical Proceedings of the Children's Hospital, Washington, D.C.,* vol. 26, pp. 97-103.

KULCZYCKI; L. L., ROBINSON, M., and BERG, C. (1969), 'Somatic and psychological factors relative to management of patients with cf', *Clinical Proceedings of the Children's Hospital, Washington, D.C.,* vol. 25, pp. 320-4.

LANGSLEY, D. G. (1961), 'Psychology of a doomed family', *American Journal of Psychotherapy,* vol. 15, pp. 531-8.

LAWLER, R. H., NAKIELNY, W., and WRIGHT, N. (1966), 'Psychological implications of cystic fibrosis', *Canadian Medical Association Journal,* May, vol. 94, pp. 1043-6.

LAWSON, D. (1965), *Cystic Fibrosis*. (pamphlet produced for parents by the Cystic Fibrosis Research Trust, Bromley, Kent).

LAWSON, D. (1971), 'A Pediatrician's Comments on the Development of Thanatology in Relation to CF', position paper to Atlantic City Symposium, April.

LEONARD, C. O., CHASE, G. A., and CHILDS, B. (1972), 'Genetic counseling: a consumer's view', *New England Journal of Medicine*, vol. 287, no. 9, pp. 433-9, August.

LEVY, D. M. (1945), 'Psychic trauma of operations in children and a note on combat neurosis', *American Journal of the Diseases of Children*, vol. 69, pp. 7-25, January.

LEWIS, M. (1962), 'The management of parents of acutely ill children in the hospital', *American Journal of Orthopsychiatry*, vol. 32, pp. 60-6.

LINDEMANN, E. (1944,54), 'Symptomatology and management of acute grief', *American Journal of Psychiatry*, vol. 101, p. 141.

LINDSAY, M., and MacCARTHY, D. (1974), 'Caring for the Brothers and Sisters of a Dying Child', in Burton, L. (ed.), *Care of the Child Facing Death*, Routledge & Kegan Paul, London.

MacCARTHY, D. (1957), 'Mothers in a children's ward', *Public Health*, vol. 71, p. 264.

MacCARTHY, D. (1969), 'The repercussion of the death of a child', *Proceedings of the Royal Society of Medicine*, vol. 62, no. 6, p. 549, June.

MacCARTHY, D., LINDSAY, H., and MORRIS, I. (1962), 'Children in hospital with mothers', *Lancet*, vol. 1, p. 603.

McCOLLUM, A. T. (forthcoming), *C.F.: Economic Impact upon the Family*.

McCOLLUM, A. T., and GIBSON, L. E. (1970), 'Family adaptation to the child with cystic fibrosis', *Pediatrics*, vol. 77, no. 4, pp. 571-8, October.

McCOLLUM, A. T., and GIBSON, L. E. (1971), Correspondence, *Pediatrics*, vol. 78, no. 3, p. 549, March.

McCOLLUM, A. T., and SCHWARTZ, A. H. (forthcoming), *Social Work and the Mourning Parent*.

McCRAE, W. M., CULL, A. M., BURTON, L., and DODGE, J. (1973), 'Cystic fibrosis: parents' response to the genetic basis of the disease', *Lancet*, July 21, pp. 141-3,

MILLER, M. L. (1951), 'The traumatic effect of surgical operations in childhood on the integrative functions of the ego', *Psychoanalytic Quarterly*, vol. 20, p. 77.

MITCHELL, M. (1973), 'Bereaved children', in Varma, V. (ed.), *Stresses in Children*, University of London Press, pp. 57-72.

MORRISSEY, J. (1963), 'Children's adaptation to fatal illness', *Social Work*, pp. 81-8, October.

MORROW, R. S., and COHEN, J. (1954), 'The psycho-social factors in muscular dystrophy', *Journal of Child Psychiatry*, vol. 3, no. 1, pp. 70-80.

MURSTEIN, B. E. (1960), 'The effect of long-term illness of children on the emotional adjustment of parents', *Child Development*, vol. 31, pp. 157-71.

NAGY, M. H. (1948), 'The child's theories concerning death', *Journal of Genetic Psychology*, vol. 73, pp. 3-27, September.

NAGY, M. H. (1959), 'The child's view of death', in Feifel, H. (ed.), *The Meaning of Death*, McGraw-Hill, New York, pp. 79-99.

NATTERSON, J. M., and KNUDSON, A. G. (1960), 'Observations concerning fear of death in fatally ill children and their mothers', *Psychosomatic Medicine*, vol. 22, p. 456.

O'CONNOR, G., and KNORR, N. J. (1968), 'Acute Trauma from a Psychological Viewpoint', in W. Ballinger (ed.), *The Management of Trauma*, Saunders, Philadelphia.

ORBACH, C. E., SUTHERLAND, A.M., and BOZEMANN, M. F. (1955), 'Psychological impact of cancer and its treatment', *Cancer,* vol. 8, pp. 20-33.

PEARSON, G. H. J. (1941), 'Effect of operative procedures on the emotional life of the child', *American Journal of Diseases of Children,* vol. 62, p. 716.

PINKERTON, P. (1969), 'Managing the psychological aspects of CF', *Arizona Medicine,* vol. 26, pp. 348-51.

PLANK, E. N., CAUGHEY, P. A., and LIPSON, M. S. (1959), 'A general hospital care program to counteract hospitalism', *American Journal of Orthopsychiatry,* vol. 29, p. 94.

POLLOCK, G. H. (1962), 'Childhood parent and sibling loss in adult patients', *Archives of General Psychiatry,* vol. 7, pp. 295-305.

PRUGH, D. G., STAUB, E. M., SANDS, H. H., KIRSCHBAUM, R. M., and LENIHAN, S. E. (1953), 'A study of the emotional reactions of children and families to hospitalization and illness', *American Journal of Orthopsychiatry,* vol. 23, p. 70.

REICHENBERG HACKETT, W. (1953), 'Changes in Goodenough Drawings after a gratifying experience', *American Journal of Orthopsychiatry,* vol. 23, pp. 501-15.

RILEY, I. D., SYME, J., HALL, M. S., and PATRICK, M. J. (1965), 'Mother and child in hospital. Two years experience', *British Medical Journal,* vol. 2, p. 990.

ROBERTSON, J. (1952), *A Two Year Old Goes to Hospital* (film), Tavistock Clinic, London; University Film Library, New York.

ROBERTSON, Joyce (1965) 'Mother-Infant Interaction from Birth to Twelve Months. Two Case Studies', in Foss, B. M. (ed.), *Determinants of Infant Behaviour,* Methuen, London.

ROGERS, R. (1966), 'Children's Reactions to Sibling Death', *Psychosomatic Medicine: Proceedings of the First International Congress of the Academy of Psychosomatic Medicine. Spain. Excerpta Medica,* International Congress Series, no. 134.

ROSENBLATT, B. (1969), 'A young boy's reaction to the death of his sister', *Journal of the American Academy of Child Psychiatrists,* vol. 8, no. 2, pp. 321-5.

ROSENSTEIN, B. J. (1970), 'Cystic fibrosis of the pancreas: impact on family functioning', in Debuskey, M. (ed.) (1970).

SAUNDERS, C. (1969), 'The management of fatal illness in childhood', *Proceedings of the Royal Society of Medicine,* vol. 62, no. 6, p. 550.

SCHAFFER, H. R., and CALLENDER, W. M. (1959), 'Psychologic effects of hospitalization in infancy', *Pediatrics,* vol. 24, p. 528.

SCHOELLY, M. L., and FRASER, A. (1955), 'Emotional reactions to muscular dystrophy', *American Journal of Physical Medicine,* vol. 34, pp. 119-23.

SHERWIN, A. C., and McCULLY, R. S. (1961), 'Reactions observed in boys of various ages to a crippling, progressive and fatal illness (muscular dystrophy)', *Journal of Chronic Diseases,* January, pp. 59-68.

SOLNIT, A. J., and GREEN, M. (1963), 'Pediatric Management of the Dying Child. II. A Study of the Child's Reaction to the Fear of Dying', in Solnit, A. J. and Provence, A. J., *Modern Perspectives in Child Development,* International Universities Press, New York, p. 217.

SOLZHENITSYN, A. (1968), *One Day in the Life of Ivan Denisovich,* Penguin, Harmondsworth.

SPENCE, J. C. (1946), *The Purpose of the Family: A Guide to the Care of Children,* National Children's Home, London.

SPENCE, J. C. (1947), 'The care of children in hospital', *British Medical Journal,* vol. 1, p. 125.

SPENCE, J. C. (1951), 'The doctor, the nurse, and the sick child', *American Journal of Nursing,* vol. 51, p. 14.

SPOCK, A., and STEDMAN, D. J. (1966), 'Psychologic characteristics of children with cystic fibrosis', *North Carolina Medical Journal*, pp. 426-8, September.

STACEY, M., DEARDEN, R., PILL, R., and ROBINSON, D. (1970), *Hospitals, Children and their Families*, Routledge & Kegan Paul, London.

STOTT, D. H. (1958), 'The social adjustment of children', manual to the *British Social Adjustment Guides*, University of London Press.

STOTT, D. H., and SYKES, E. H. (1956), *British Social Adjustment Guides*, University of London Press.

TEICHER, J. D. (1969), 'Psychological aspects of cystic fibrosis in children and adolescents', *California Medicine*, vol. 110, no. 5, pp. 371-4.

TILL, M. M., HARDISTY, R. M., and PIKE, M. C. (1973), 'Long survivals in acute leukaemia', *Lancet*, pp. 534-8, March 10.

TISZA, V. B. (1960), 'Management of the parents of the chronically ill child', *American Journal of Psychology*, vol. 32, pp. 53-9.

TROPAUER, A., FRANZ, M. N., and DILGARD, V. (1970), 'Psychological aspects of the care of children with cystic fibrosis', *American Journal of Diseases of Children*, vol. 119, May.

TURK, J. (1964), 'Impact of cystic fibrosis on family functioning', *Pediatrics*, pp. 67-71, July.

VAUGHAN, G. F. (1957), 'Children in hospital', *Lancet*, vol. 1, p. 1117.

VISOTSKY, H. M., HAMBURG, D. A., GOSS, M. E., and LEBOVITS, B. Z. (1961), 'Coping behaviour under extreme stress. Observations of patients with severe poliomyelitis', *Archives of General Psychiatry*, vol. 5, p. 423.

WAECHTER, E. H. (1968), 'Death Anxiety in Children with Fatal Illness' (unpub. doctoral dissertation), Stanford University.

WALKER, J. H., and THOMAS, Russell (1971), 'Spina bifida and the parents', *Developmental Medicine and Child Neurology*, vol. 13, pp. 462-76.

YUDKIN, S. (1967), 'Children and death', *Lancet*, p. 37, January 7.

Author index

Subject index

Printed and bound by CPI Group (UK) Ltd, Croydon, CR0 4YY

17/10/2024

01775680-0004